THIS IS THE PICTURE

The drug free approach to dealing with Depression, Anxiety, Stress, Low Self-Esteem, Anger, Drugs and Alcohol Addiction. This book includes self-help exercises and is suitable for anyone who is keen to deal with life's modern day illnesses without the use of drugs and medication.

Written by Paul Burton and

produced by Melanie Jane Milligan.

This Is The Picture

Published by
Chipmunkapublishing
PO Box 6872
Brentwood
Essex CM13 1ZT
United Kingdom

http://www.chipmunkapublishing.com

Edited by Mary Dew

Chipmunkapublishing gratefully acknowledge the support of Arts Council England.

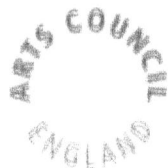

INTRODUCTION

The aim of this book is to help everybody who reads it to develop a clear insight into common mental health disorders.

Throughout my years of experience working in mental health, I have realised that most people who are depressed struggle to find the motivation and concentration required to follow a self-help book. With this in mind I have created a simple-to-follow, colourful illustrated book that carefully guides the reader through all of the main points that they will ever need to know.

Accompanying the illustrated sections is a more detailed text that the reader can chose to dip in and out of whenever they require a more detailed explanation, or when they are feeling better able to concentrate. Each section of the book is accompanied by a series of easy-to-follow exercises that gradually build up into a fully comprehensive treatment plan.

I hope that this will book will prove to be a useful tool in the fight against depression and mental illness.

(Paul Burton = 2004)

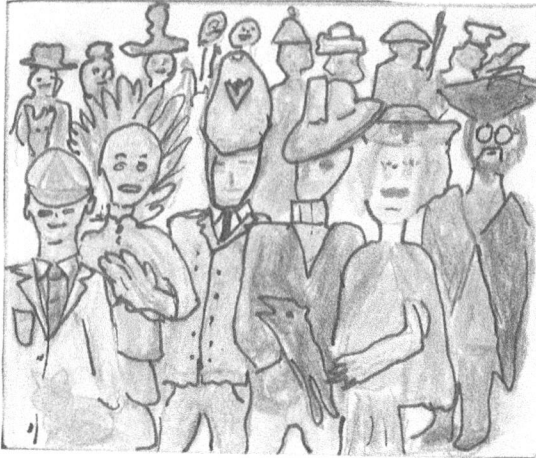

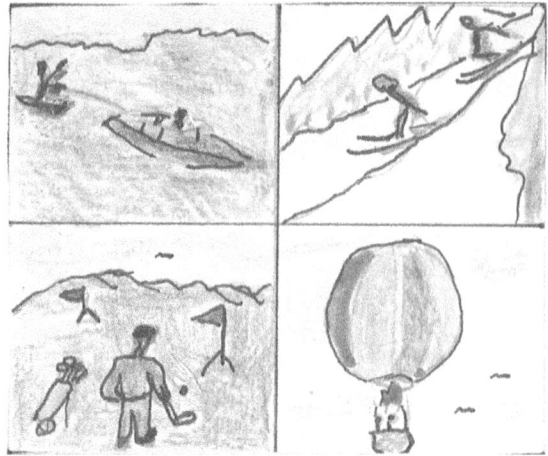

This book is designed to help everybody.		It should help you to make the most out of your life.

WHO SHOULD READ THIS BOOK?

This book is designed to help absolutely everyone. It is not purely aimed at people who are currently suffering from mental health problems, such as anxiety and depression. It is also designed to help people prevent the onset of depression and mental illness, and to enable everyone that reads it to make the most out of their lives, whether they are currently unemployed or are the managing director of a major company.

In short, it is a recipe book for life, a guide to help you avoid a lot of the pitfalls that threaten us all. A book that will help you to get to know yourself, and to understand yourself enough to know exactly what you want to get out of life. It will give you the necessary skills needed to plan and execute a path to your full potential so that you can enjoy your life to the full.

The advice laid out in this book relates to all of us without exception, so keep it on your coffee table or next or your bed. Take your time reading and digesting the information in it, because this book could not only change your life, it could also save your life!

ANXIETY

DRUGS AND ALCOHOL

STRESS

DEPRESSION

ANGER

LOW SELF-ESTEEM

POOR ASSERTIVENESS

It is a very lucky man who
avoids all of the traps,
For the traps are plentiful
and dangerous.

Yet the man who learns how to escape
from the traps is luckier still,
For he now has insight and wisdom
to guide him.

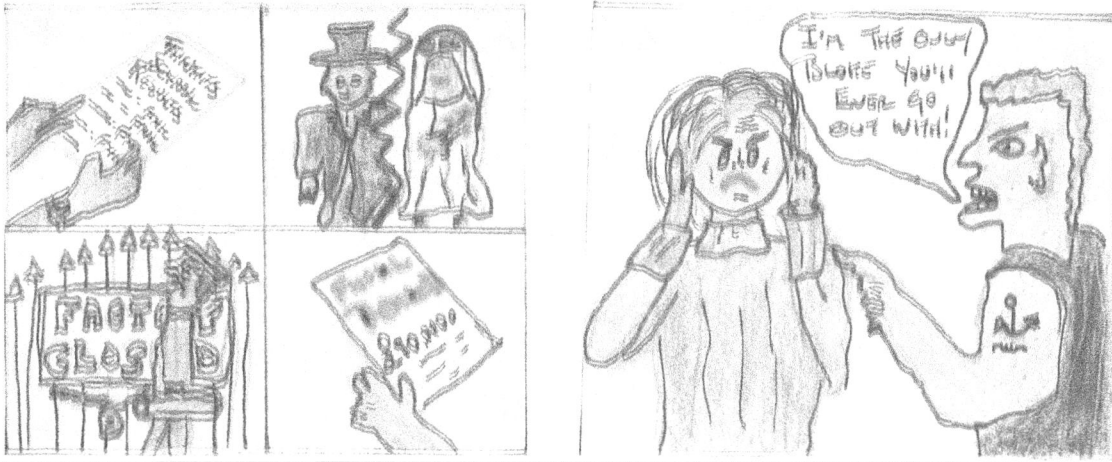

Many life experiences can cause depression.		If we understand the cause, we are more likely to be able to change things.

SOME POSSIBLE CAUSES OF DEPRESSION.

There can be many reasons why any one of us can start to feel depressed. Here are some of the most common causes of depression:

- Recent bereavement of a close family member or friend.

- Long-term poor physical health/caring for somebody with poor health.

- Coming to the end of a close loving relationship.

- Feeling lonely and unloved

- Ongoing disputes at work or at home.

- Unemployment/poor job prospects/feeling trapped in a rut.

- Financial worries/debts/poverty/accommodation problems.

- Having no sense of meaning or purpose to our lives.

- Sexual problems/sexual identity problems.

- Being a victim of crime/injustice/racism/sexual harassment.

- Parental difficulties.

- Struggling to deal with an addiction/loved ones' addiction.

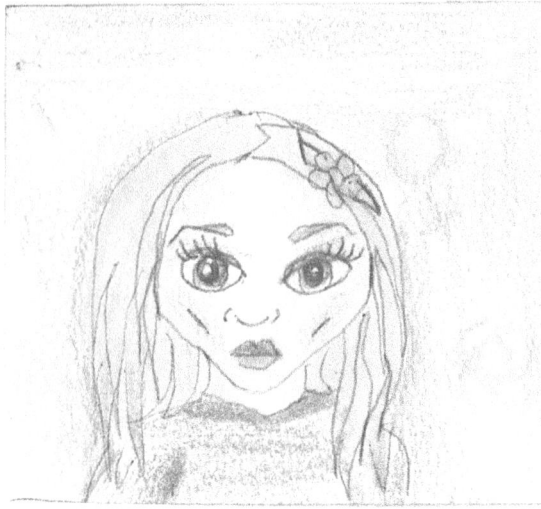

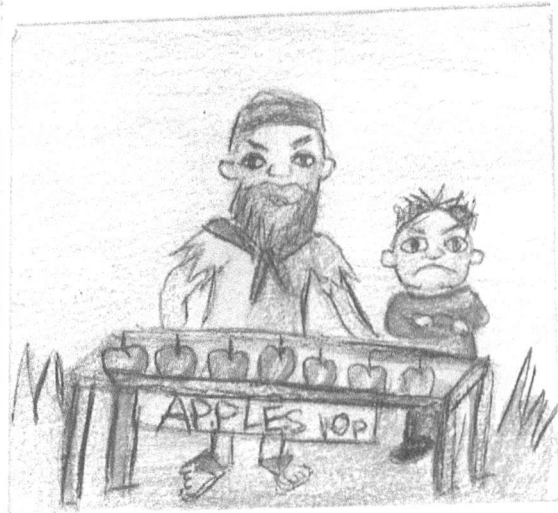

Females are more likely than males to suffer from depression.		Poor people are more likely to get depressed.

SO WHO IS MOST LIKELY TO SUFFER FROM

DEPRESSION?

Although depression knows no boundaries and upsetting life events can happen to anyone of us at any time in our lives, there are a few groups of people who are far more likely than others to be affected by reactive depression.

- Poverty is one determining factor; if we are poor we are more likely to be inundated with unpleasant life events. We will be more susceptible to stress and ill health, along with low self-esteem as we struggle to cope with poor working conditions and exploitation. We will also lack the funds to engage in pleasant pastimes that could counteract stress.

- Being female increases your chances particularly after childbirth.

- Having a family history of depression or other mental health conditions will increase your chances of developing a depressive illness.

Now do Exercise 1.

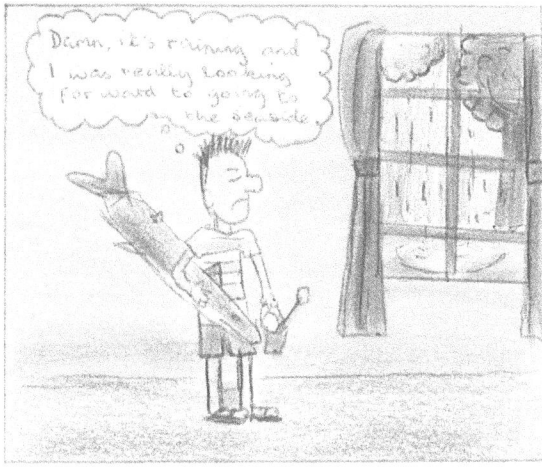

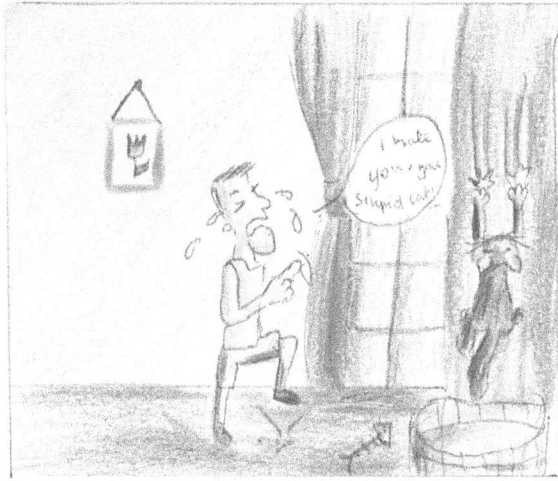

It is easy to misinterpret feeling sad for depression.		It is perfectly natural to sometimes feel unhappy or sad.

JUST WHAT IS DEPRESSION?

Defining depression is a very difficult task because we are all so different. The symptoms can vary enormously from person to person according to each individual's own set of unique personality traits, and the different ways that each of us tends to perceive things. We all get fed up, sad and disgruntled from time to time, but these feelings are natural and don't necessarily mean that we are becoming depressed. It is only when these feelings persist for an unnaturally prolonged length of time and then start to affect our ability to function normally, that depression can truly be considered as a possible diagnosis.

Unfortunately, once we believe that we are suffering from depression, we can enter into a very difficult and prolonged illness that will fuel itself. Ironically, we only ever seem to get better once we tell ourselves that we are no longer suffering from depression.

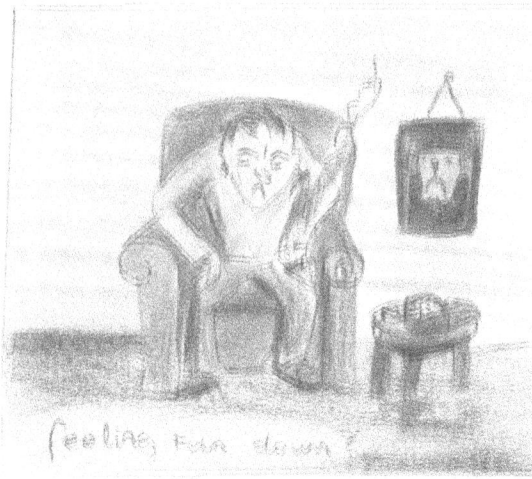

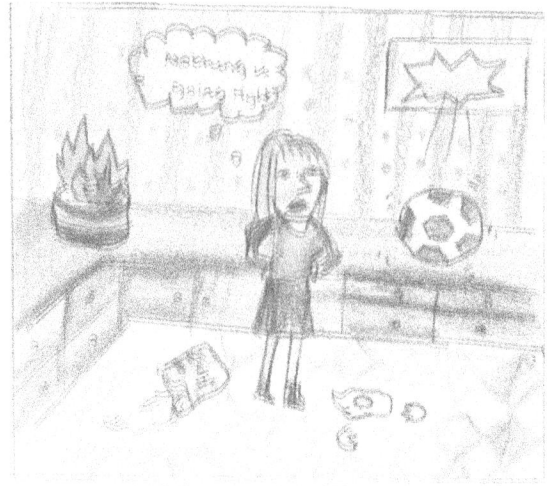

It is easy to start feeling fed up and disgruntled.		Nothing seems to go right.

THE SYMPTOMS OF DEPRESSION.

It is very common to feel fed up and disgruntled with everything, nothing seems to have any relevance or importance anymore, we can feel removed from life, often feeling like an outsider watching life go by. Tasks like daily chores and cleanliness can start to be disregarded, as we no longer see any point in carrying them out. It feels like a major effort is required to carry out the simplest of tasks and when we do attempt to perform them they never seem to go to plan. So we become even more frustrated with ourselves, which in turn increases our inner feelings of helplessness and failure. We end up giving up on our lives and ourselves as we fail to recognise the importance, value or significance of anything.

We may well develop further problems such as low self-esteem and a lack of assertiveness and confidence. We may become very anxious or maybe very angry. We might even develop a dependency upon drugs or alcohol.

Now do Exercise 2.

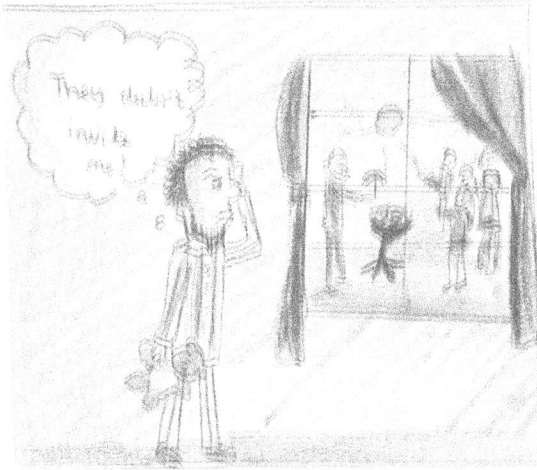

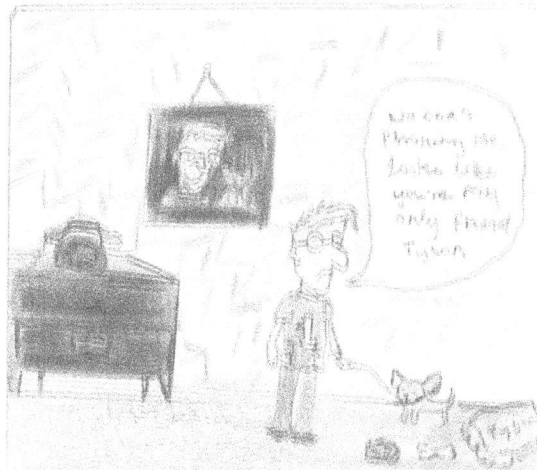

We can start to feel that other people don't want to know us.	We may start to cut ourselves off from the outside world.

THE CIRCLE OF DEPRESSION.

Unfortunately not many of us are very good at dealing with somebody who is constantly low in mood and depressed. Most people want to be able to have a good laugh when going out with their friends. Yes, some old friends will be there for us in the early stages of depression, but as time goes by, more and more people will avoid us. This is because they do not want to be brought down by our negativity, and they will probably have already tried everything that they can think of in order to cheer us up, and now they no longer know what they can possibly do. So avoidance soon becomes the easiest answer for them.

We interpret this as rejection, and so our feelings of worthlessness and depression continue to increase, along with new feelings of loneliness and isolation.

Now do Exercise 3.

15

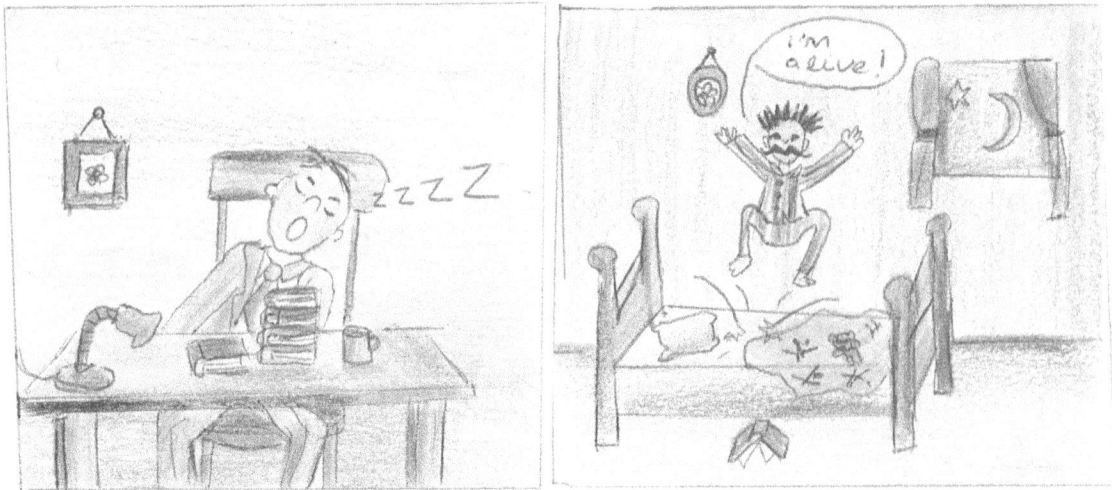

Some people sleep too much.		Some people cannot sleep at all.

THE SYMPTOMS OF DEPRESSION CAN VARY A LOT.

Some people find that depression changes their sleeping habits. Lack of sleep can, in a very short space of time, impair your ability to concentrate, affect your ability to problem solve and reduce your capacity to make rational decisions. It can also make you irritable and short-tempered. So just imagine how damaging lack of sleep can be if it persists for many weeks! Is it any wonder that depressed people often struggle to concentrate or make a decision about anything?

Recent studies have also concluded that when we sleep our minds sort out our problems for us, a bit like a magic filing cabinet that puts everything into it's proper place. If we are unable to do this our thinking becomes seriously impaired and we may get easily confused, lowering our mood even further. On the other hand, too much sleep can make you slow and lethargic, tasks are put off and our lack of enthusiasm for anything increases our feelings of depression even more.

Now do Exercise 4.

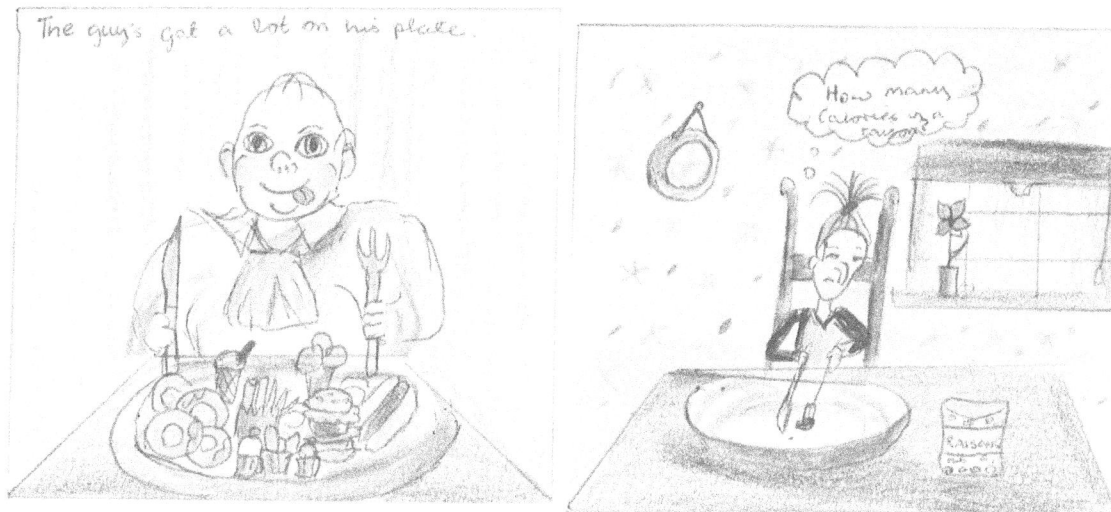

Some people eat too much.		Some people struggle to eat anything at all.

DEPRESSION CAN AFFECT OUR EATING HABITS.

Depression often affects sufferers' eating habits; some people find that they no longer want to eat, while others find it difficult to stop eating. We all need to eat in order to keep our bodies working; food is our fuel, just like petrol is a car's fuel. If you have no petrol in your car it is unable to move. Sometimes running out of fuel can also damage other parts of the car that have struggled to function without it. If we stop putting fuel into our bodies it can have a similar effect. Not only are we starving ourselves of essential vitamins and minerals, we are preventing our bodies from being able to fight back naturally against illness because the extra energy required is simply not there. We also become weak and susceptible to picking up other illnesses, lowering our mood even further.

If we over eat we start to gain weight, which in turn makes exercise even harder so we become lazy and lethargic, our self-esteem and confidence go down as we start to hate the way that we now look. It is therefore important to maintain a regular, healthy balanced diet at all times.

Now do Exercise 5.

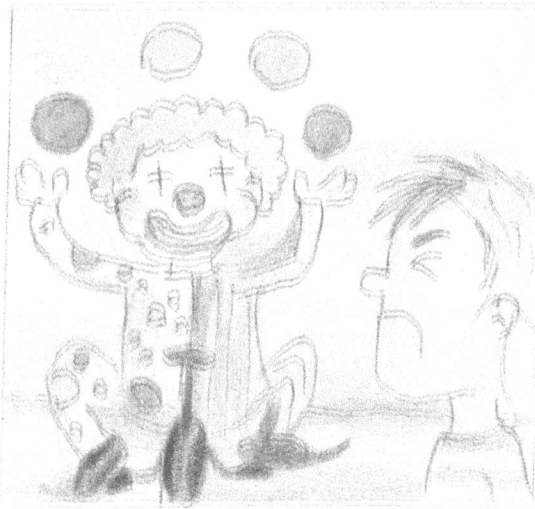

| Some depressed people find it hard to show any emotion at all. | Some become over emotional. |

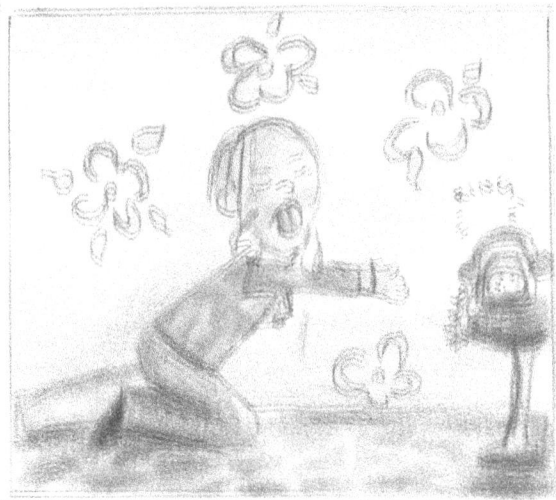

OUR EMOTIONS CAN START TO CHANGE.

A lot of people tend to see depression purely as an illness of the emotions and although emotions play a large part in the case of most depressions, they are certainly not the only symptom. It is however fair to say that suffering from depression can cause havoc with our emotions. Sufferers of depression can often become over emotional, often crying at the smallest of things or sometimes crying without understanding what it is that they are crying about. Some sufferers can get very angry, while others struggle to show any emotion at all about anything. No matter what happens good or bad, they find it very difficult to show any enthusiasm or emotion, as they seem to have reached a point where they are past caring about anything anymore.

We are usually very good at keeping a lid on our emotions and hiding our true feelings from the outside world, but depression breaks down this control mechanism, exposing us to our true raw feelings and emotions.

Now do Exercise 6.

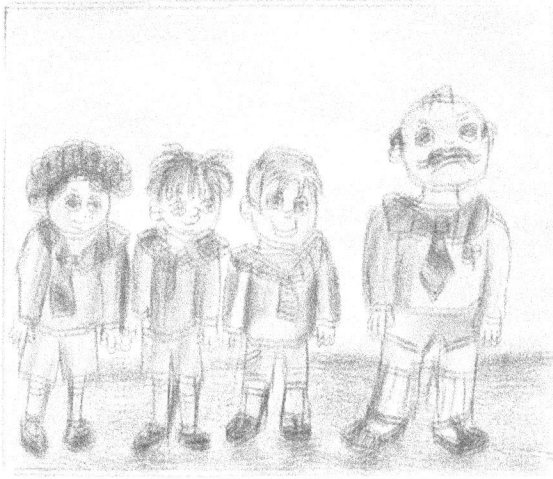

We can lose interest in things we used to enjoy.		As time goes on it can become harder to get motivated.

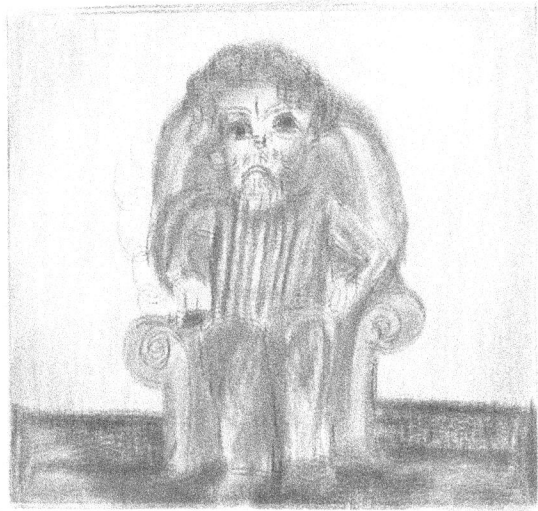

INTEREST AND MOTIVATION SEEM TO DESERT US.

One of the hardest things for us to deal with when we are feeling depressed is our complete loss of interest in things. Sometimes things that we used to enjoy doing now seem pointless and boring. Nothing seems to be of any value or importance any more, so there seems to be very little point in trying to do anything at all, and the less that we do the harder it becomes to find any motivation. This eventually leads us to a situation where we are so unmotivated that even if we do find something that we really would like to do we are now no longer motivated enough to be able to do it. This leads to us spending more and more of our time just sitting around focusing upon how depressed we feel, which in turn leads to an increase in low mood and depression. We will have managed to trap ourselves into a negative cycle of functioning that will continue unless we manage to break the pattern ourselves.

Now do Exercise 7.

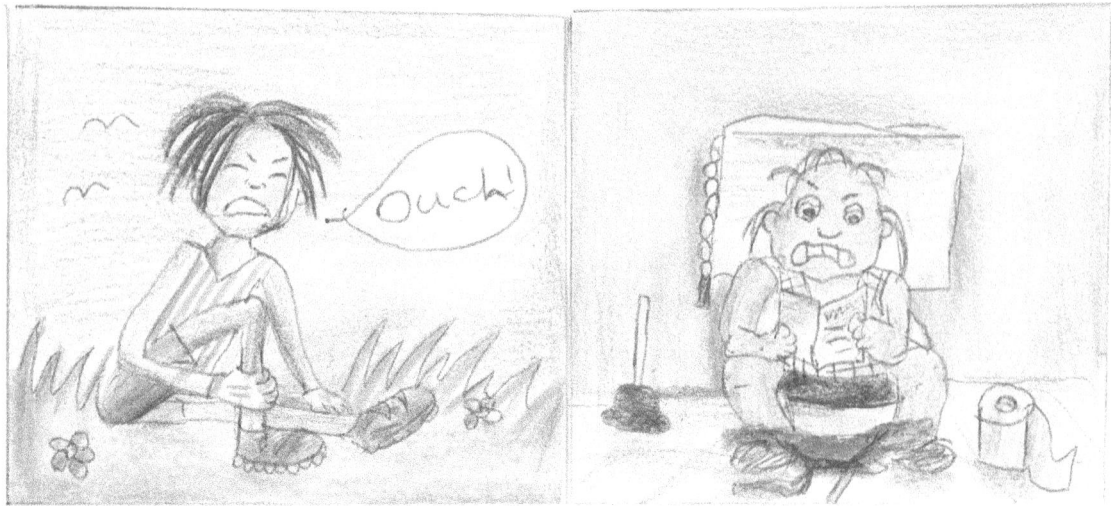

We can suffer from aches and pains.		Constipation.

DEPRESSION CAN ALSO AFFECT US PHYSICALLY.

Depression is not just an illness of the mind; it can also have some quite marked physical effects upon us as well. Common difficulties include:

- Headaches

- Digestive problems

- Skin complaints / acne

- Weight loss / weight gain

- Loss of libido

- Insomnia

- Constipation

- General aches and pains

Of course we cannot put all our physical complaints down entirely to depression but we can be pretty sure that they are associated with the fact that our immune system is very run down. Again we find ourselves trapped into a negative cycle as suffering from these conditions starts to make us feel even more depressed.

Now do Exercise 8.

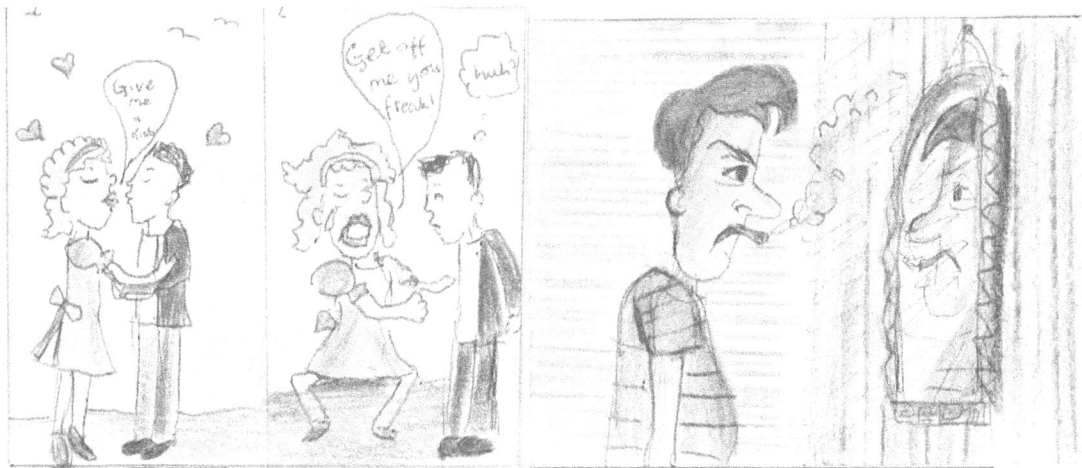

Depression can affect the way that we behave towards each other.	We can start to hate ourselves or who we have become

DEPRESSION CAN ALSO AFFECT OUR BEHAVIOUR.

It is quite common for us to actually start hating ourselves when we become depressed. We can feel that we no longer like the person that we see in the mirror. We can start to over analyse every aspect of our own behaviour and because we are already feeling very negative, we can find ourselves being over self-critical. We may start to relive past events in our minds over and over again, but none of these will be happy events, instead we will focus upon negative unpleasant events. Events where we behaved badly or foolishly will tend to haunt us so much that we start to regard ourselves as dreadful unworthy people. This in turn will affect the way that we come across to others, making them very wary and cautious of us, which will have the knock-on effect of increasing our negative beliefs about ourselves, thereby increasing our own feelings of depression.

Now do Exercise 9.

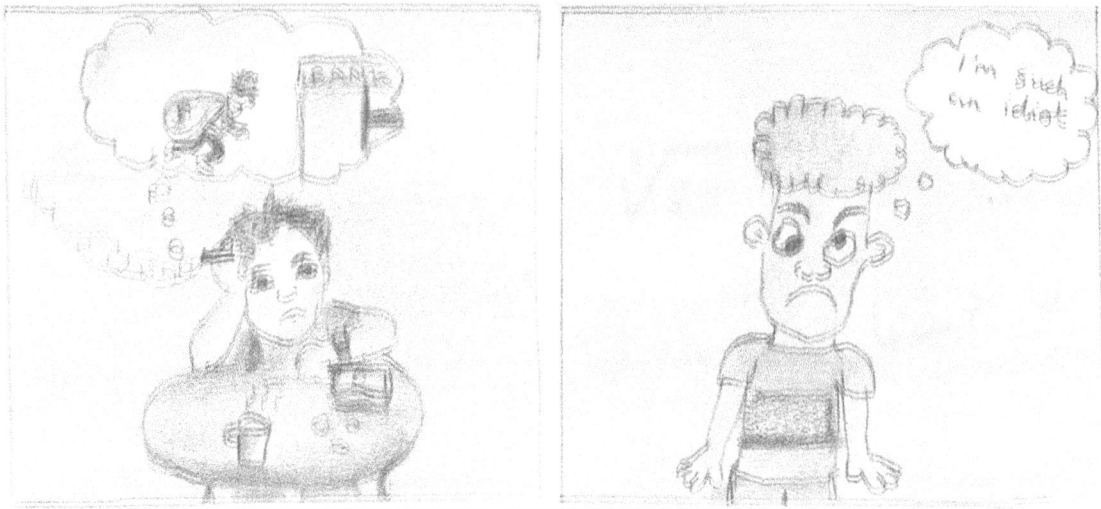

We can start to feel guilty and worthless.		We can start to develop a low opinion of ourselves.

OUR OPINION OF OURSELVES CAN GO DOWN.

We can start to feel that all of the problems of the world are in some way connected to us and that everything is our fault. Although we rationally realise that this cannot be true, in our minds at the time it seems like a perfectly reasonable conclusion. This leads to us feeling incredibly guilty about ourselves. We start believing that we must in some way be a really bad and worthless person. Such feelings then come out when we communicate with others and they pick up on it treating us accordingly. This increases our negative feelings and lowers our self-esteem even further, which in turn increases our feeling of depression.

Now do Exercise 10.

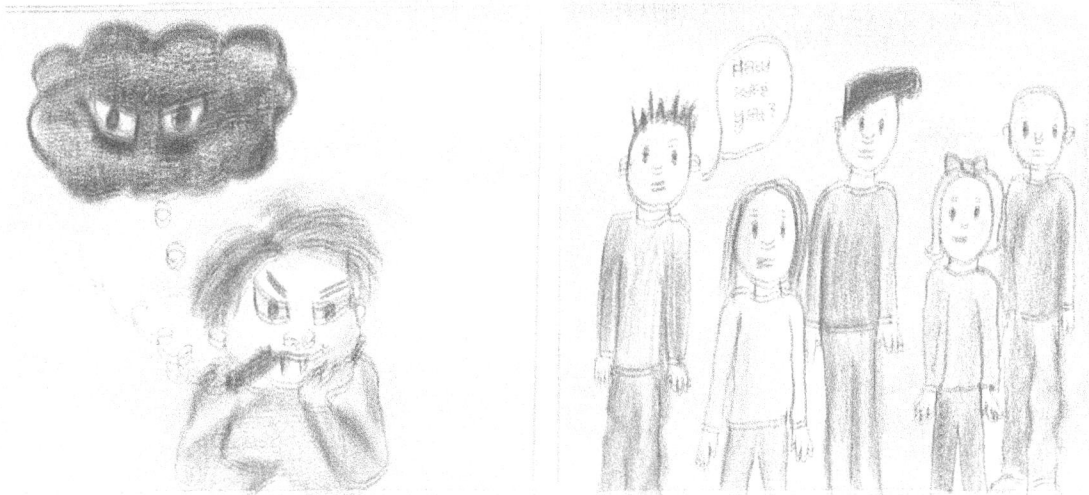

We can experience dark bleak thoughts.		We may feel that everyone is watching us.

DARK, DEPRESSING THOUGHTS CAN TAKE OVER.

Sometimes we can start to suffer from dark intrusive thoughts; we might experience bleak disturbing images in our minds of things that would never normally occur to us. This can be a very disturbing and upsetting experience, but it is really only a reflection of how low our mood has become. Other symptoms can include:

- Feeling very scared and thinking that other people are talking about us.

- Believing that people are staring and laughing about us.

- Misinterpreting things that other say to us.

These sorts of experiences are generally referred to as paranoid symptoms. Paranoid symptoms can be brought about by drug and alcohol misuse and they can also occur when we are suffering from a very high temperature, but when they start to occur for no apparent reason the chances are that they are a symptom of a mental illness.

Now do Exercise 11.

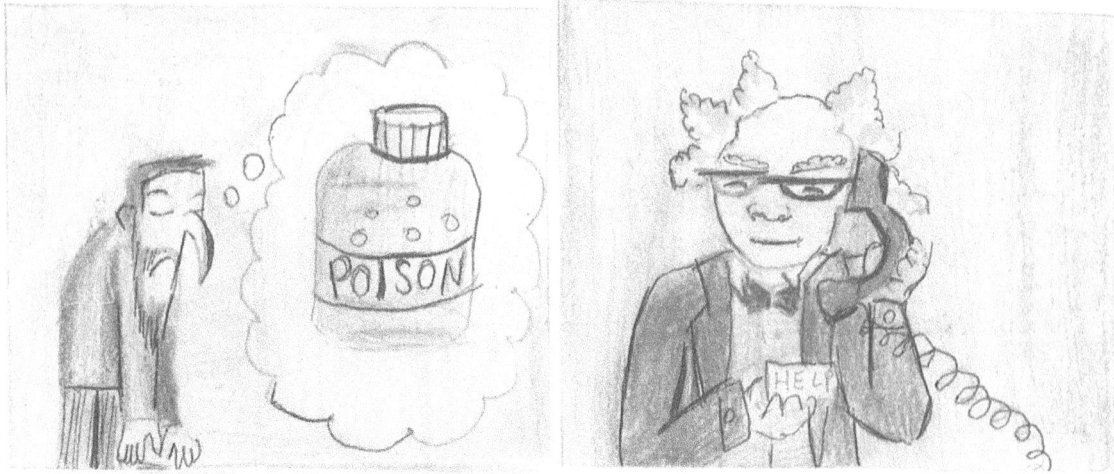

Thoughts of suicide are only a temporary state.		Seek out professional help

WE CAN BE PLAGUED BY SUICIDAL THOUGHTS.

When you combine the feelings of worthlessness with dark intrusive thoughts, it is little wonder that a lot of people start to feel that life is no longer worth living and so they might consider suicide as a viable option. At the time suicide probably appears to be the only possible way out of the very desperate situation that they find themselves in. Once any of us have reached this state, the probability is that we are unable to think clearly about anything anyway.

Most people that have contemplated suicide at a certain point in their life, later realise that it was a very desperate and dangerous time for them, but they are now pleased that they did not carry it out because life moves on and changes do happen. If you are ever feeling suicidal you must remember that the crisis you currently find yourself in is only a temporary state, in a short space of time you will be looking back with relief that you did not carry it out.

Now do Exercise 12.

24

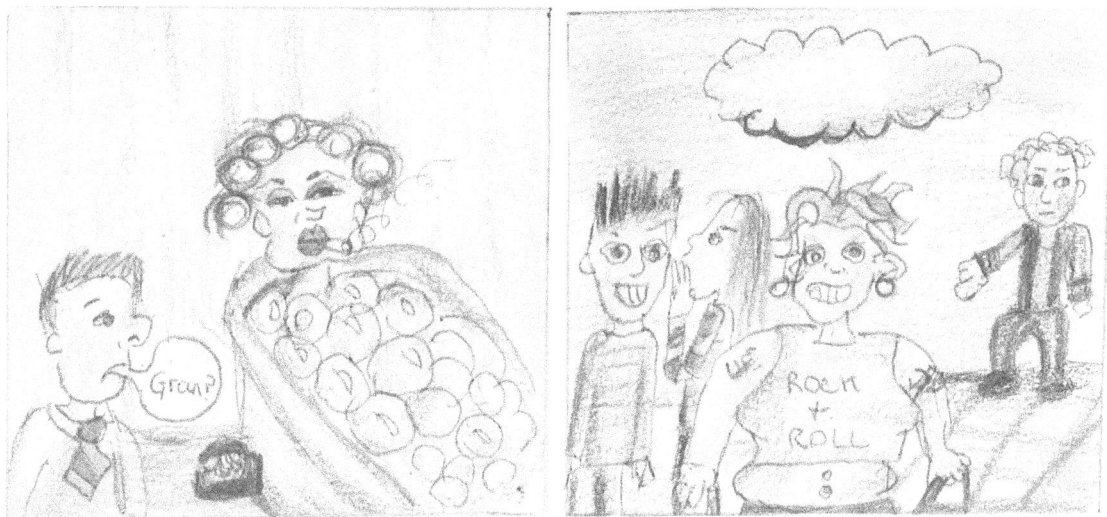

Sometimes we can lose all track of time.		We might turn up somewhere at an inappropriate time.

OUR SENSE OF TIME CAN BECOME AFFECTED.

Depression can affect our sense of time and punctuality. We can often miss appointments or turn up somewhere at completely the wrong time of day. This can happen for a number of reasons:

- Our body clock may be completely out due to poor sleeping patterns

- Our memory may be badly impaired by depression

- We might continuously be deeply entrenched in our own inward thoughts

- Our lack of motivation can make it difficult to get anywhere

- With so few other commitments it can become hard to stick to any at all

- We may no longer value some appointments due to our low mood

Now do Exercise 13.

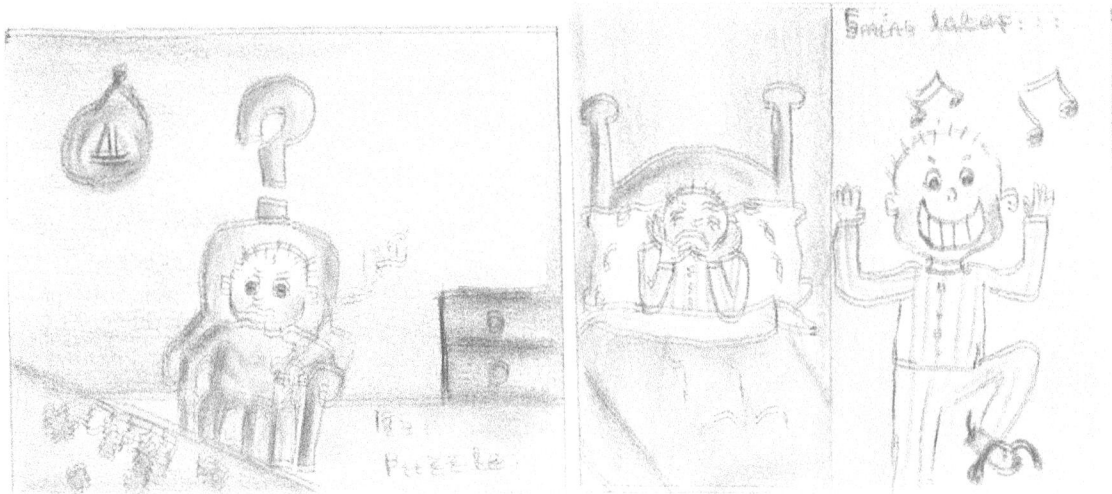

Endogenous depression seems to have no cause.		Manic depression is when you suffer from extremes of mood.

SO WHAT SORT OF DEPRESSION HAVE I GOT?

There are three main different types of depression that we can suffer from.

1) **Manic Depression or Bi-Polar Disorder** is a relatively rare condition where your mood swings from a very low depressive state into a very high euphoric state. When you are in a high state you tend to believe that you are capable of absolutely anything. Some people get into debt after funding outrageous business ideas or buying things that they can't possibly afford. Others believe that they are famous historical figures and some people have so much energy that they can't stop cleaning! During a low period, sufferers tend to become socially withdrawn, physically and mentally exhausted and very low in mood. Manic depression is a very difficult condition to live with because most sufferers have no idea when their next mood swing will happen, so planning anything in advance becomes very difficult and precarious.

2) **Endogenous Depression** is the name given to a depression that seems to have no external cause. We know that there are chemical changes taking place in our brains when we become depressed, so it could be that chemical changes within the brain are actually causing sufferers of endogenous depression to become depressed.

26

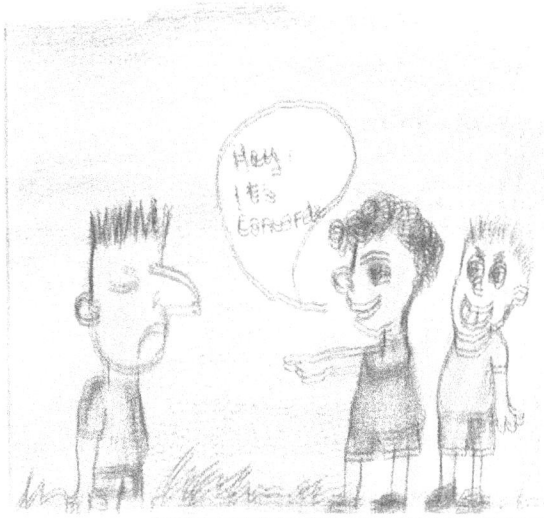

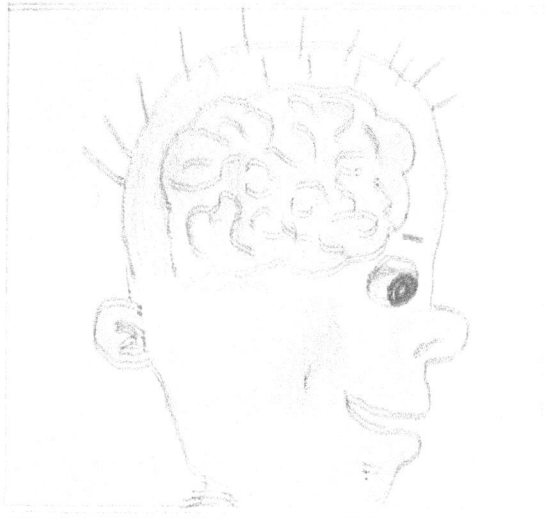

Reactive depression is a reaction to unpleasant life events.	Sustained low mood will eventually affect the chemicals in your brain.

WHAT IS A REACTIVE DEPRESSION?

3)   **Reaction Depression** is by far the most common; it will affect approximately 10% of the population at some point in their lives. It is called reactive because we are reacting to unpleasant life events by lowering our mood level. The causes of reactive depression can vary greatly from person to person depending upon our personality type, life situation, coping skills, experience and our values. As time goes on we begin to become overwhelmed by our depression, the initial trigger to our depression can often start to fade into insignificance. This is because chemical changes to our brains have already started to change the way that we now think.

Whether we are suffering from manic depression, endogenous depression, or reactive depression, the road to recovery is going to be pretty much the same for all of us. Medication may well help, but nothing is as important as really getting our life on track so that we are living the life that we want to live and doing the things that will make us happy.

Now do Exercise 14.

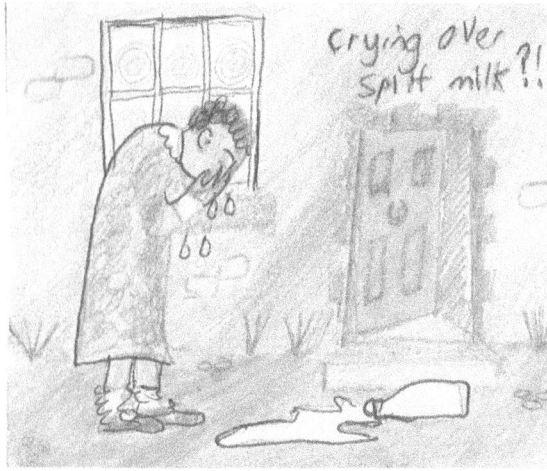

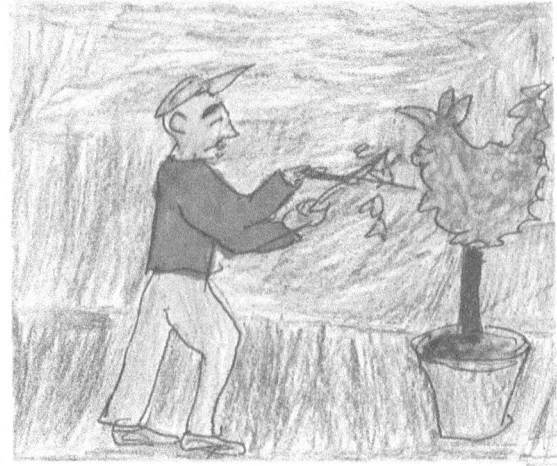

| Some conditions do require antidepressant medication. | Medication is not always the answer a pro-active approach can be very beneficial. |

DO WE NEED TO TAKE ANTI-DEPRESSANT MEDICATION?

For some of us taking medication is going to be an essential part of any treatment plan. We are going to need to take medication if:

- We are hearing voices telling us to do things that we do not want to do

- If we are experiencing visual hallucinations

- If we are experiencing overwhelming feelings that are making us feel like harming either others or ourselves

- If we are feeling so low in mood that we feel unable to make any headway or progress whatsoever

- If we are suffering from a manic or endogenous depression.

Medication can be very helpful for some people but as the symptoms of depression vary so much it is often very difficult to find the right medication to fit our individual needs. In general it is either going to have a relaxing effect upon us or it is going to give us a bit more drive to do things. The trouble is that medication on it's own is rarely the answer and it should never be seen as such. Making positive changes to our lives that help us to feel better about ourselves, is a far more affective approach then just taking a pill and waiting for changes to happen. There is also the problem that every time that we take a pill we remind ourselves that we are still suffering from depression.

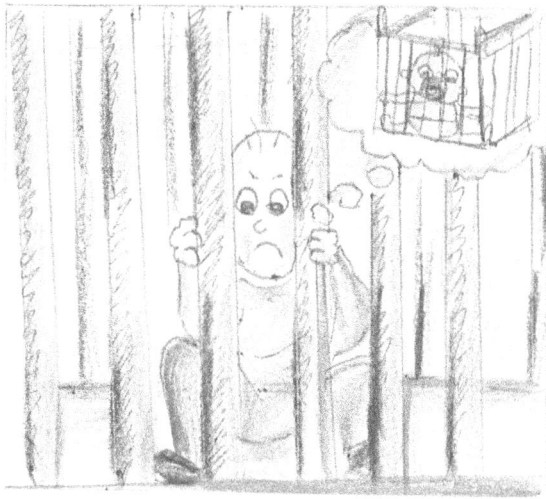

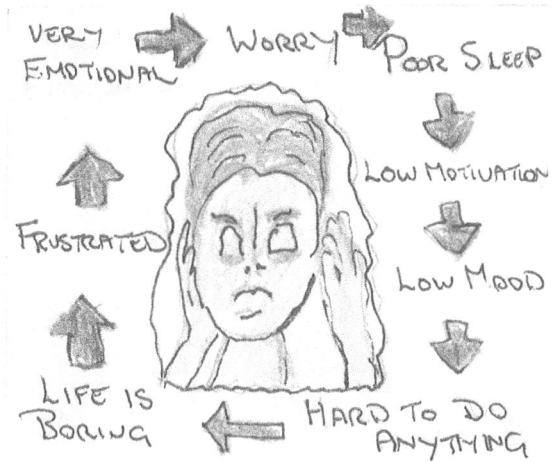

We can easily become very trapped by our symptoms.		Each symptom tends to fuel the next symptom.

DEPRESSION CAN BECOME A SELF-PERPETUATING DOWNWARD SPIRAL.

Most of the symptoms that we suffer from with depression do tend to fuel each other and so we easily end up becoming stuck in a self-perpetuating circle of dysfunction. For example:

- Our appearance starts to decline due to depression

- We feel self-conscious and ashamed about our appearance

- So we start to lose our self-confidence

- We no longer have the confidence to try anything new

- We become stuck in the same old routine that made us depressed

- Being depressed makes us neglect our appearance

This is just one example of how easily we can become trapped in our own cycle of depression. This is why so many people find it so difficult to ever escape from their depression.

Now do Exercise 15.

It is a very lucky man who avoids all

of the traps,

For the traps are plentiful and dangerous,

Yet the man who learns how to escape from the

traps is luckier still,

For he now has insight and wisdom to

guide him.

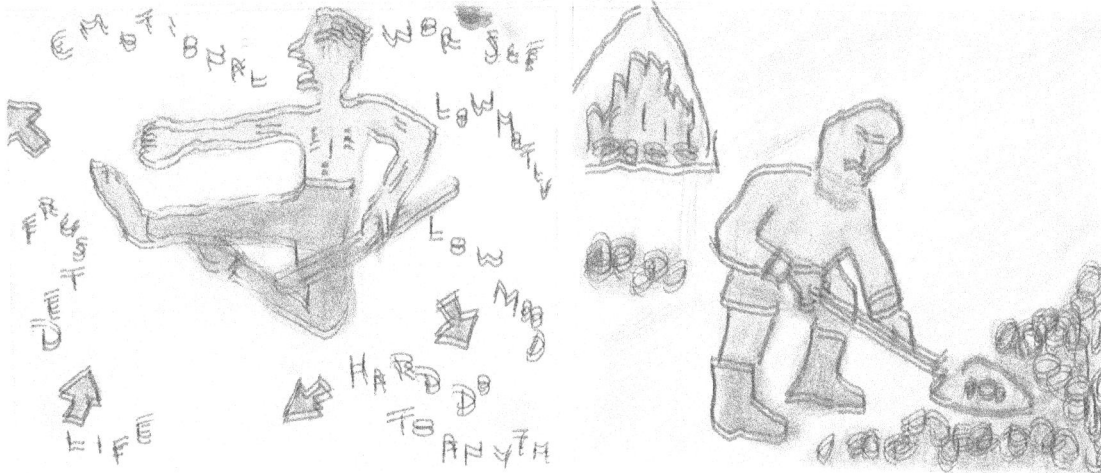

Breaking the negative cycle is to going to be difficult.		Are you prepared to work hard in order to get better?

IMPROVEMENT CAN ONLY COME FROM WITHIN.

As we have just seen the symptoms of depression keep fuelling each other and when that affects our motivation, our concentration and our energy levels it becomes a very difficult cycle to break out of. Added to this is the fact that society also seems to be contributing to our negative cycle by making it very difficult for us to return to fully paid employment. Then by making dependence upon the welfare state seem like a far safer option than independence, we soon realise that conquering depression once it has taken over our lives is going to be a very tough and difficult battle. Nonetheless, it certainly is possible to conquer depression if you can find the willpower and motivation to keep on track.

The first step that we have to make is to tell ourselves that we are totally committed to conquering depression no matter what it takes. Once we have made this decision we will be firmly established on the road towards recovery.

Now do Exercise 16.

31

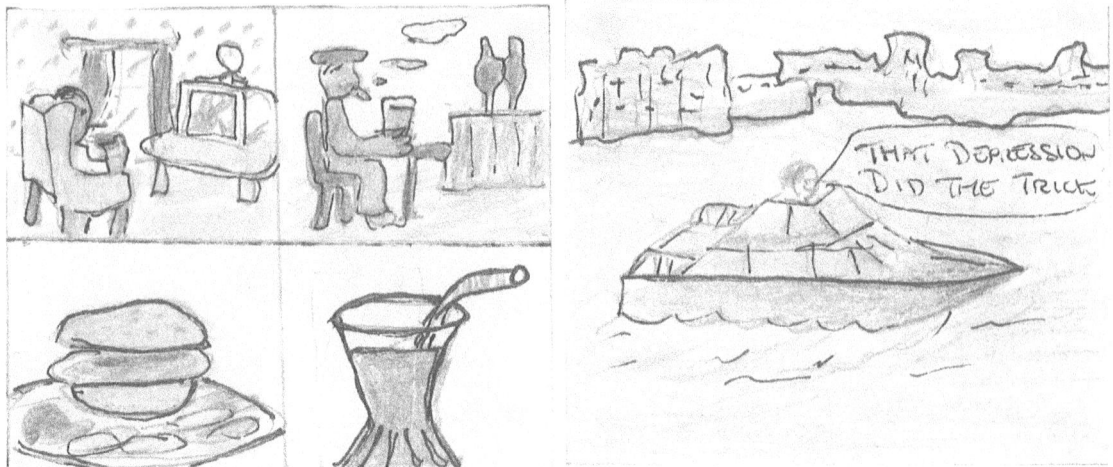

Depression might have been caused by your lifestyle to date.		Try to see depression as a positive thing that will eventually improve your life.

WHAT DO YOU WANT TO HAPPEN?

In order for us to improve we need to have a clear idea of what improvement means to us. How will we know when we are better? What needs to happen before we can say that we are no longer depressed? It is always easier for us to get somewhere when we know where it is that we want to go. A vague idea about feeling better is not really enough to guide us. We need to accept that our depression probably happened because we needed to make some changes to ourselves and to our lives. If we fail to make any changes then we will become stuck in an ongoing depression, but hopefully in years to come we will be able to look back upon our depression in a new positive light. Ultimately seeing it as a major turning point in our life that brought about a lot of positive and beneficial changes. It is after all a learning experience, even if it does seem very unpleasant at the time.

If we can start to view depression in this new light, then we can start to generate positive changes in our thinking and attitude that will help us to eventually conquer depression for good.

Now do Exercise 17.

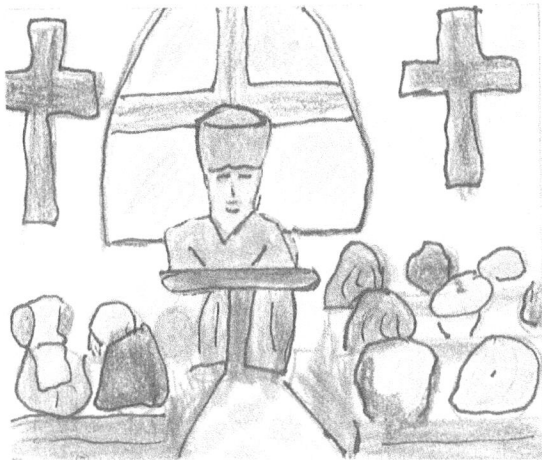

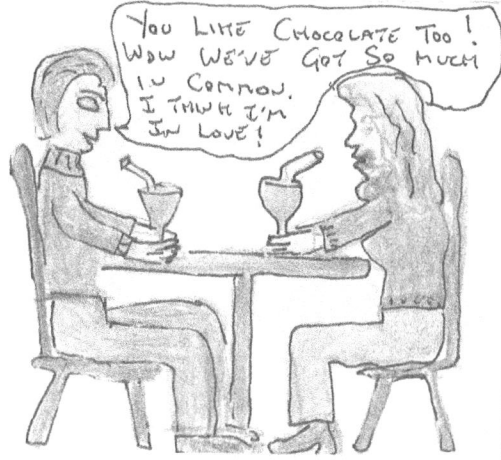

Having beliefs gives us an identity.		Relationships are built upon shared beliefs.

WHAT DO WE REALLY BELIEVE IN?

Beliefs can take many forms and cover a vast range of topics, they are important because they are what we choose to represent us. If we put on a football shirt we are immediately identified as somebody who supports that football team. If we attend a particular church we are identified as somebody who believes in that religion. So our beliefs are the building blocks of our identify. Whenever we meet somebody new, the first thing that we tend to subconsciously do is to look for some kind of common ground. "What sort of music do you like? What sports do you follow?" Once we have found some shared beliefs we can go on to form a relationship with that person. If we fail to identify any shared beliefs, the relationship will not develop any further because it will lack any foundation to build upon. When we meet somebody that we really want to bond with, we often try to discover as much as possible about his or her beliefs, so that we can find some common ground in which to cement the relationship. Sometimes we are so in love that we are willing to adopt some of their beliefs, just so that they will accept us.

Now do Exercise 18.

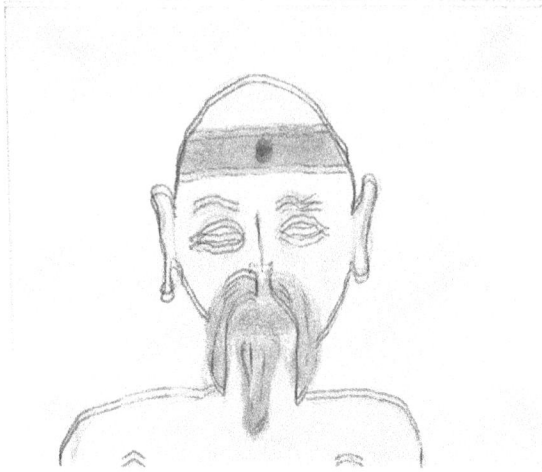

We need to think deeply about what we really believe in.	Going against our beliefs creates inner conflict.

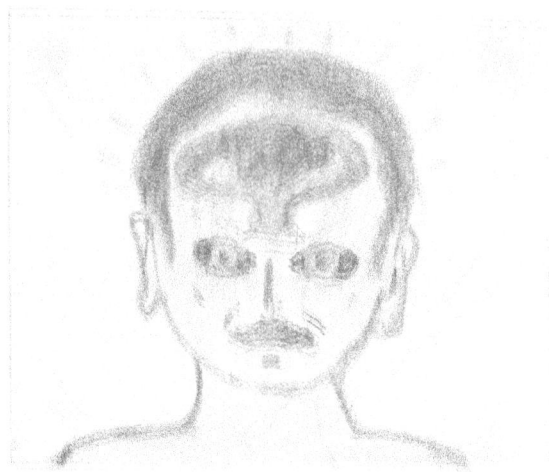

WE NEED TO RE-DISCOVER OUR BELIEF SYSTEM.

During an episode of depression we can become very inward looking and a lot of our previously held beliefs can start to seem irrelevant and meaningless. We need to use this situation to our own advantage by digging deep inside ourselves and doing some major soul searching. Only then can we can start to find out what our true beliefs really are. If we can then incorporate our beliefs into the treatment plan that we are gradually devising for ourselves, our chances of successfully conquering depression will greatly increase because we will be doing the things that we really believe in.

It is only when we find ourselves going against our beliefs that we create inner conflict and dissatisfaction. Our beliefs can and do change over time, so we need to acknowledge this in order to keep in line with them, we also need to be able to change and adapt with them, so that we remain in harmony with ourselves.

Now do Exercise 19.

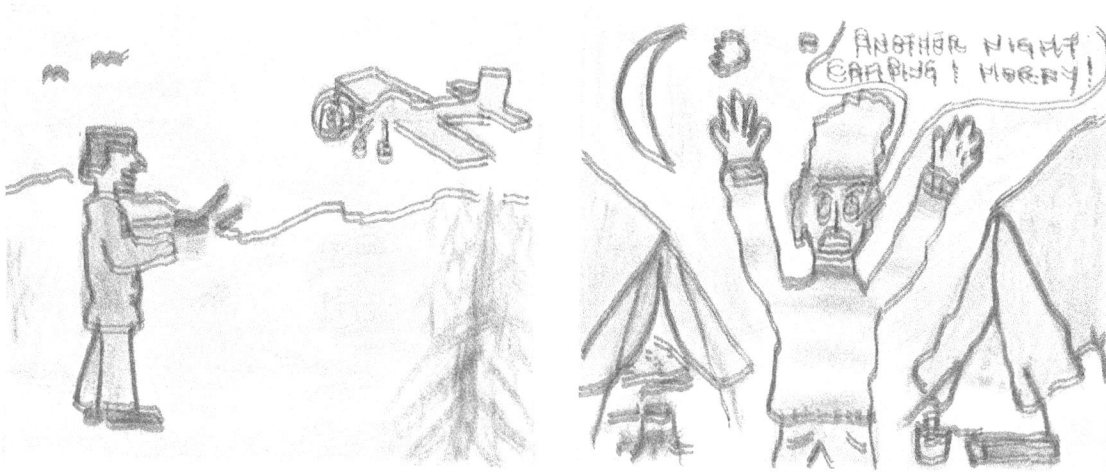

We can value meaningless things that bring us pleasure.		When we value what we do our enthusiasm rises.

WHAT ARE VALUES ABOUT?

Whereas a belief is a firmly held opinion, our values are more of a judgement about the things that we have found to be important in life to us. We may not have a belief about water skiing, but we might still place a high value upon having the time and the resources to participate in it as often as possible. So values are quite different from beliefs. We can value things that are fairly meaningless yet tend to bring us pleasure, whereas our beliefs do not necessarily bring us any personal satisfaction but they do act as a moral guiding force. If we can find some value in the things that we do, our enthusiasm rises and we tend to put in a far better performance. When we perform better our self-esteem rises making us value ourselves more, which in turn reduces feelings of depression.

So if we have a clear idea about what we value, we can use that information to guide our recovery by focusing more upon activities that we value, rather than activities that we find unfulfilling.

Now do Exercise 20.

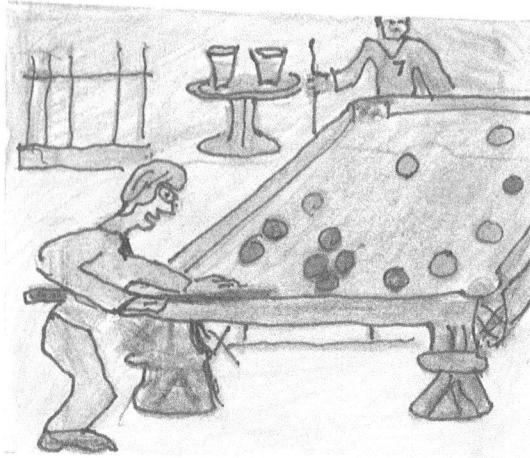

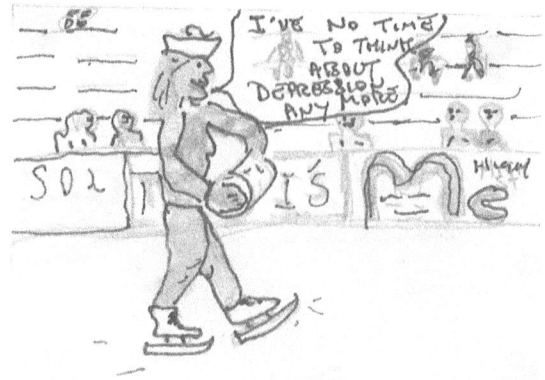

Interests are the things that we choose to do.		Interests can prevent us from developing depression.

WHAT ARE INTERESTS AND WHY DO WE NEED THEM?

Interests are very important because they are the things that we choose to do with our own time. So much of our lives are taken up with chores and tasks that we do not choose to do but have to do in order to survive. Interests are the things that we don't have to do at all. They should therefore bring us a lot of fulfilment, satisfaction, and enjoyment. If they don't then you might be pursuing the wrong interests. Having interests is also a very important preventative measure against us developing depression in the first place because interests help us to maintain concentration, improve our memory and increase our drive and enthusiasm. Some interests also improve physical fitness and stamina, along with providing us with a social network of friends who are not solely connected to work. Interests always work better for us when they incorporate some of our beliefs and values into them. So for example if you believe that fresh water fishing is morally justifiable and you value the opportunity to eat fresh fish, it stands to reason that you may be able to fully immerse yourself into the hobby of fishing.

Now do Exercise 21.

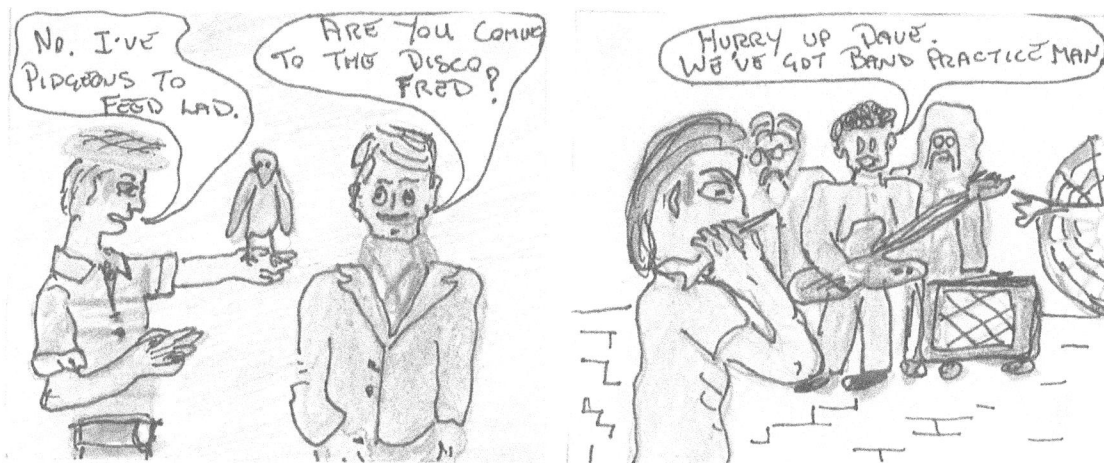

Our interests gradually change as we grow older.		When we are depressed we need interests more than ever.

OUR INTERESTS CHANGE OVER TIME.

As we grow older our interests gradually change, we may not be fit enough to pursue the same sports any more so we replace them with less physically demanding ones. We may develop new interests like pottery or gardening as we gradually move away from old interests like disco dancing or skate boarding. This is a very natural progression that happens so gradually to most people that they barely notice it. Unfortunately when we are depressed we tend to drop interests very rapidly due to our loss of motivation and interest. We tend not to replace these interests for the same reasons - and so the very things in life that used to bring us happiness, meaning and satisfaction have now gone, just when we need them the most!

It would be far better if we could increase the time that we spend pursuing our interests when we are starting to feel depressed, rather than decreasing it. We all need to learn to value and respect our leisure time.

Now do Exercise 22 by completing the table at the back of the book.

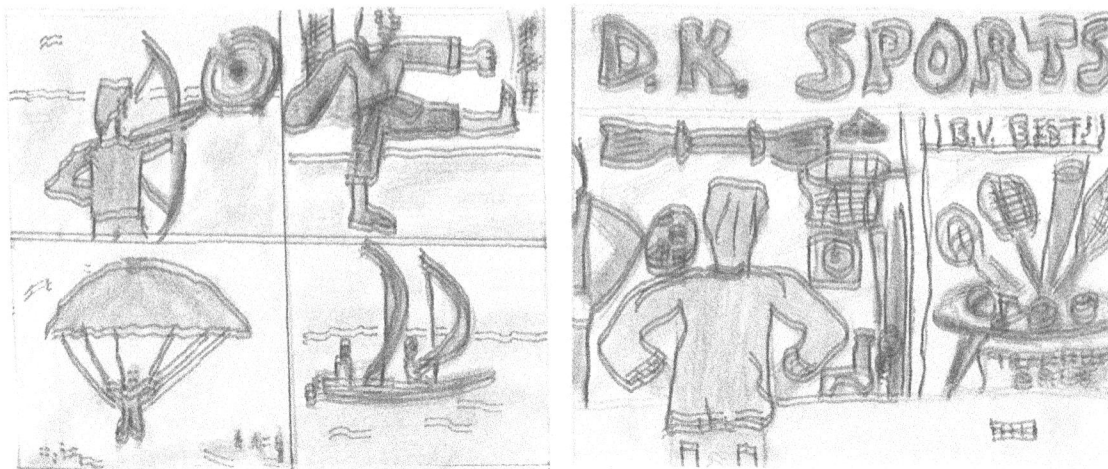

Identify some interests that you wish to pursue.		Make some positive plans to start a new interest.

WHAT YOUR CHART ACTUALLY MEANS.

For most people suffering from depression the past column will normally contain the most ticks, whilst the present column will contain the least. This is because we have gradually lost our enthusiasm and motivation for past interests. The all-important column is the future one. Hopefully we can add more ticks to that than the present column because we need to identify some interests that we would like to pursue in the future. If we haven't managed to add any ticks to the future column, then we need to focus upon what we would be doing with our time if we felt well because it is vital that we tick some boxes in this column. Once we have identified some interests that we would like to pursue in the future, we can start to incorporate them into our treatment regime as long-term goals. If we have managed to identify some new interests that we would like to pursue in the future, then we can congratulate ourselves because we are already adopting a new, far more positive outlook on life and this will definitely aid our recovery.

Now do Exercise 23.

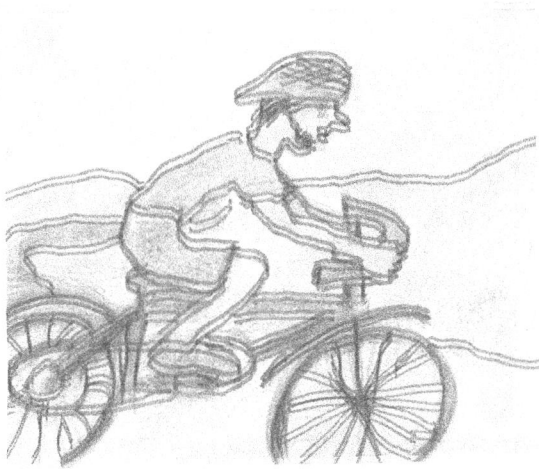
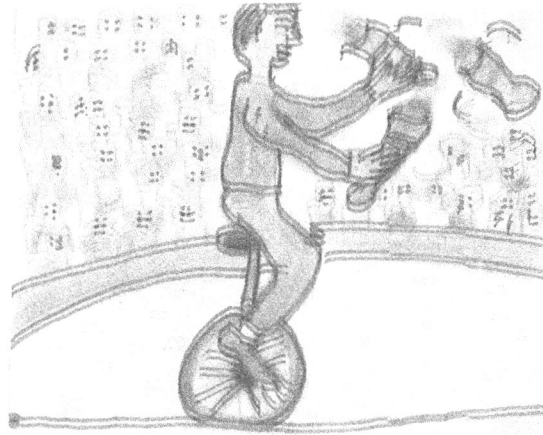

| Interests can help us to improve upon our level of functioning. | Identify some interest that could improve your level of functioning. |

USE INTERESTS TO IMPROVE FUNCTIONING.

Different activities require different skills. If we can identify which skills we are currently experiencing problems with then we can find some suitable activities that require us to use those skills. The more that we use our skills, the greater the improvement in our functioning will be. It is however not always obvious just which skills are required to perform certain tasks. It is not until you really start to analyse some tasks in details that you realise just how beneficial some activities can be. For instance cycling requires balance, co-ordination, stamina, hand-eye-co-ordination, strength, focus, information processing, concentration and planning. Judo requires planning, physical strength, stamina, awareness, balance, co-ordination, focus and teamwork. Art requires hand-eye co-ordination, imagination, memory, information processing, vision, creativity and planning.

Now do Exercise 33.

39

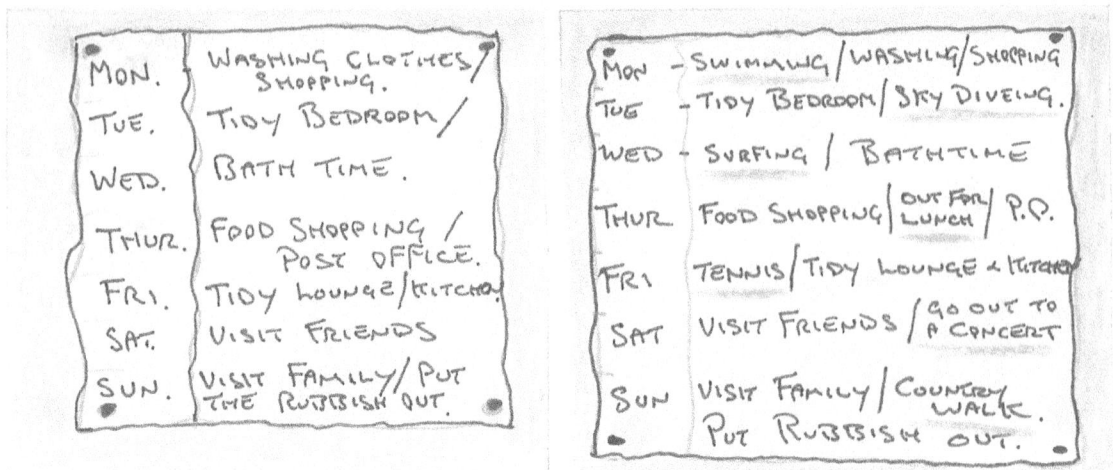

List all of the tasks that you have to do each week.		Include pleasurable activities and times for relaxation.

EFFECTIVE TIME MANAGEMENT.

Time management is not just for highflying businessmen, we all need to be able to organise our time as effectively as possible. Ironically it seems that the more time that we have to fill, the less organised and productive we become. When we are depressed, it becomes even more vital to manage our time effectively because apart from suffering from poor motivation, lack of enthusiasm, and low energy levels, the last thing that we want to be doing is sitting around all day just thinking about how depressed we have become. You should by now have a list of interests that you intend to pursue. You will also have many other essential tasks that you need to do on a daily or weekly basis in order to survive. These include tasks like washing, cleaning, shopping, cooking and eating. When we fail to carry out these essential tasks our feelings of self-loathing and failure increase, making us feel even more depressed. This is why constructing a simple timetable is so helpful as well as useful. If we list all of the tasks that we need to carry out each week giving equal importance to work, rest and play activities, then we can use this information to construct a timetable and use it to regain some control over our lives.

Now study the example at the back of this book and do Exercise 25.

40

Left timetable:

	9am	10am	11am	12	1pm	2pm	3pm	4pm
MON		WASH		TIDY ROOM	LUNCH		READ	
TUE		SHPP	SHOP		LUNCH	TIDY BATHROOM		
WED		WALK	RELAX	LUNCH				Read
THUR	WASHING			LUNCH		READ		SHOP
FRI		TIDY LOUNGE			LUNCH		HOOVER HALL	
SAT		Read		LUNCH		SHOP	SHOP	
SUN		WALK	RELAX		LUNCH		READ.	

Right timetable:

	9am	10am	11am	12	1pm	2pm	3pm	4pm
MON	JOGGING	WALK	RELAX	TIDY Rm.	LUNCH	WASH UP	READ	
TUE	SWIM	SHOPPING		READ	LUNCH	TIDY	TIDY	
WED	JOGGING	WALK	READ	LUNCH	READ	WASH		
THUR	WASHING	GYM	LUNCH	READ		SHOP.		
FRI	TENNIS	TIDY HOUSE		LUNCH	CLEAN CARPETS			
SAT	WALK	READING	LUNCH	SHOPPING	CINEMA			
SUN	JOG	WALK	RELAX		LUNCH	READING		

USE A TIMETABLE TO BALANCE YOUR LIFE.

The first thing that usually strikes us when we start to construct a timetable for ourselves, is just how many blank unaccounted for one hour long time slots we have left once we have filled in all of our essential tasks. Even when we add in our new interests, there still appears to be a lot of blank slots. This is in fact a good thing because it is far better for us to have a sparse timetable that we can keep to rather than a full timetable that we will struggle with and more than likely give up on. After a few weeks we can start adding to our timetable on a very gradual basis so that we become more and more active. It is best if we try to fit in a good mixture of activities each day by interspersing mundane activities between pleasurable ones and physically demanding activities between restful ones. By doing this we can learn to improve upon our stamina, our motivation, our tolerance and our concentration. Rewarding ourselves each week for keeping on task can also improve our motivation. This doesn't have to be a big reward, just something pleasurable. The beauty of this idea is that if our timetable suddenly starts to feel too demanding we don't have to totally give up on it; instead we can gradually reduce activities until we feel comfortable and able to cope again.

Now do Exercise 26.

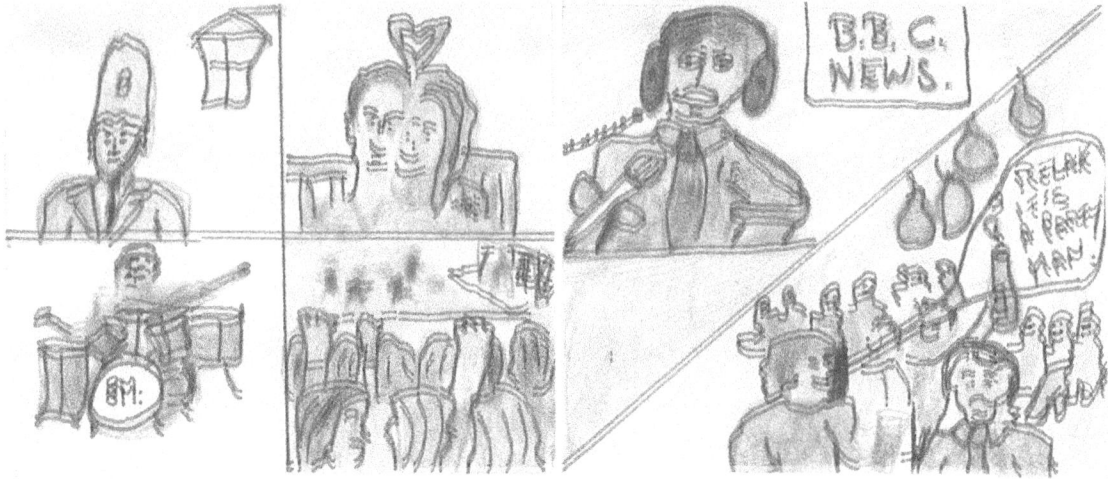

| We all behave differently according to which role we are currently in. | We can be very confident in some roles and very shy in others. |

WHAT EXACTLY ARE ROLES?

Have you ever noticed how we all change our character depending upon the situation that we find ourselves in? If you don't agree with me then just imagine yourself in the following scenario. You are in a pub with some work colleagues when suddenly your best friend comes in and joins you, then your ever-friendly rather peculiar neighbour asks if he can join you too. Next your father comes into the pub looking for you because he is keen to introduce you to your uncle whom you haven't seen for 15 years. Then your GP comes into the pub and sits right next to you. How do you feel?

Most of us would be pretty uncomfortable in this scenario because the chances are that each of these people would know a very different side of our personality to the others, and so we would feel very unsure of how we should best behave. Or to put it another way, in this scenario we would be torn between our work role, our friend role, our neighbour role, our sick role and our family role. We all change depending upon which role we are in; in some roles we can appear to be very confident and assertive, while in others we seem shy and vulnerable. We can be happy in some roles and very sad in others.

Now do Exercise 27 completing the roles identification table at the back of this book.

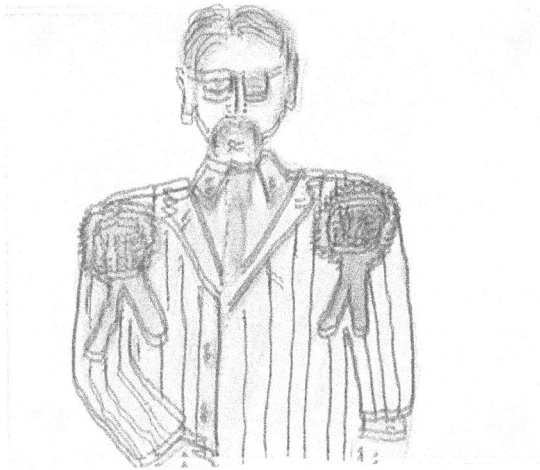

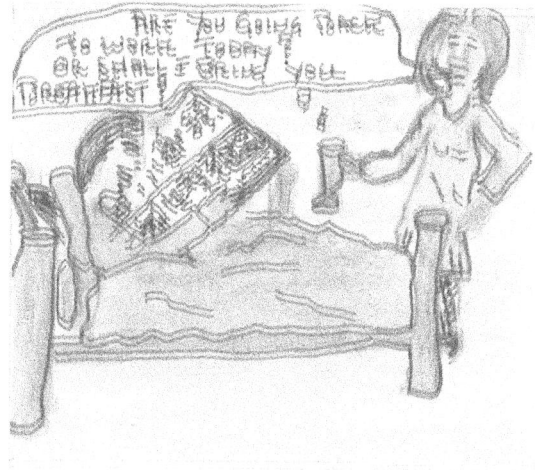

Roles help us to develop a balanced personality.		The sick role can be very difficult to break away from.

WHY ARE ROLES SO IMPORTANT TO US?

Having a variety of roles in our lives helps us to develop a sense of self-awareness, which in turn shapes our entire personality. A good balance of roles therefore allows us to develop our full potential and become balanced individuals. Too many roles can lead us to confusion over our true identity, while too few roles can prevent us from reaching our full potential, and can keep us stuck in dysfunctional situations. We all use the sick role when we are ill because it can be very beneficial for us to hand over all of our responsibilities so that we can just focus upon our own well being for a short time. We also tend to self-wallow in pity so that others will offer us sympathy and take care of us. This is fine for brief periods of illness but when it goes on for too long, as it usually does when we are depressed we can end up becoming stuck in only the sick role. This is because to us it feels like the safest place to hide, but unfortunately it is a trap the longer we stay in the sick role, the more our other roles decrease in importance and so we start to fear and avoid them.

Now do Exercise 28.

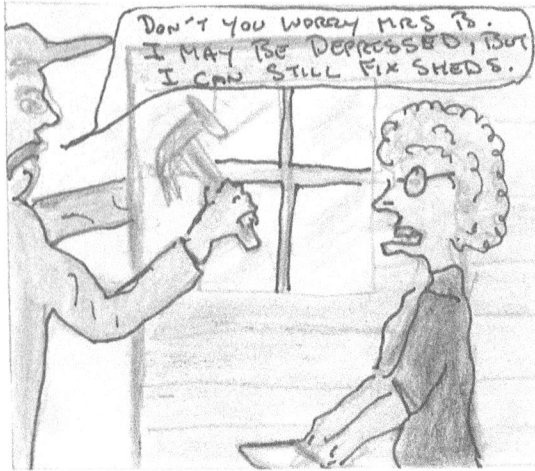

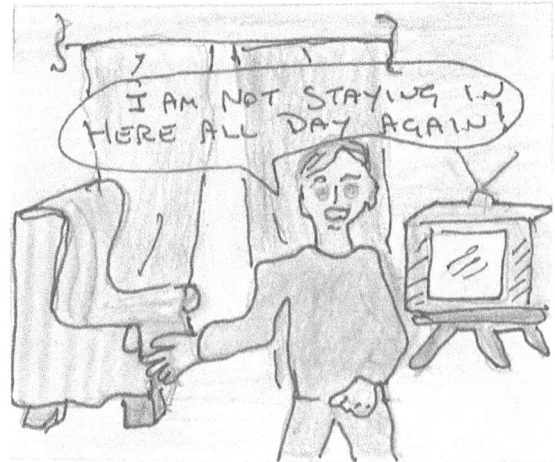

Increase the amount of time that you spend in functional roles.	Decrease the amount of time that you spend in the sick role.

BREAK OUT OF THE SICK ROLE.

After studying the list of roles most of us become quite shocked by how many roles we have now discarded due to feelings of depression. We therefore need to make some positive plans to help us to develop new roles for ourselves. We now need to analyse how we perform in each of these roles in a bit more depth, so that we can learn to use our roles to our own advantage. We need to ask ourselves which roles we feel happiest in, which roles do we feel healthiest in, which roles do we feel the most confident in and which roles make us feel low in mood? By understanding ourselves more we can learn to use our roles as a means of escape from the sick role. In order to do this we need to ask ourselves what we currently gain from being in the sick role? Do we really want to go through life with people just feeling sorry for us or would we prefer them to respect us for the person that we really are? The idea of change is frightening to all of us because we have become accustomed to the way that we are. It is almost as if we are better off with the devil that we know. But when that devil is causing us so much misery don't we owe it to ourselves to try and change?

Now do Exercise 29.

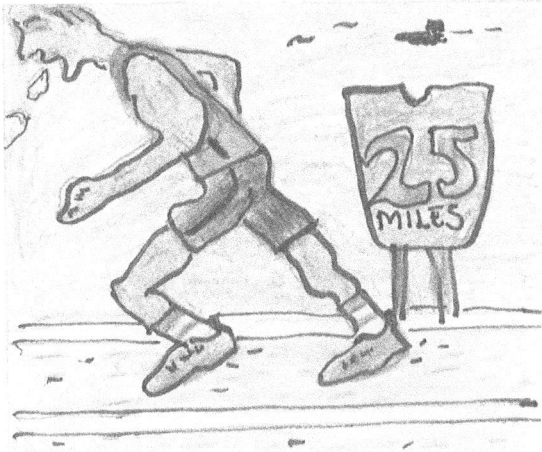

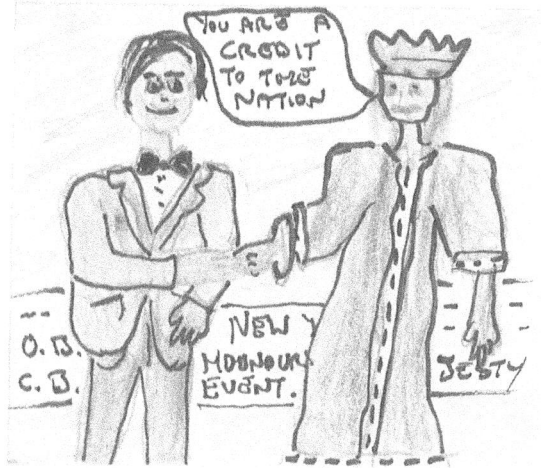

Long-term goals give us drive and determination.		We all need to aspire to achieving something that we can feel proud about.

WHY DO WE NEED GOALS?

We all need goals to aim for because they have a remarkable effect upon us. They are the driving forces that give us the energy, determination and courage to persevere and achieve.

Without ambition our lives can easily become meaningless, dull and boring. It is never too late in life to have an ambition or a long-term goal that we wish to achieve. It doesn't have to be anything amazing like climbing Mount Everest. It can be something quite basic like learning a new recipe or a card game. What the goal is doesn't really matter, what matters it that it is something that we really want to achieve because if we are not bothered about it we will never make any progress towards achieving it.

When we think of somebody going full out to achieve their ambition, we do not usually associate them with depression, yet in reality the actions that they are taking are probably fuelled by an overwhelming desire to avoid depression more than any other factor.

Now do Exercise 30.

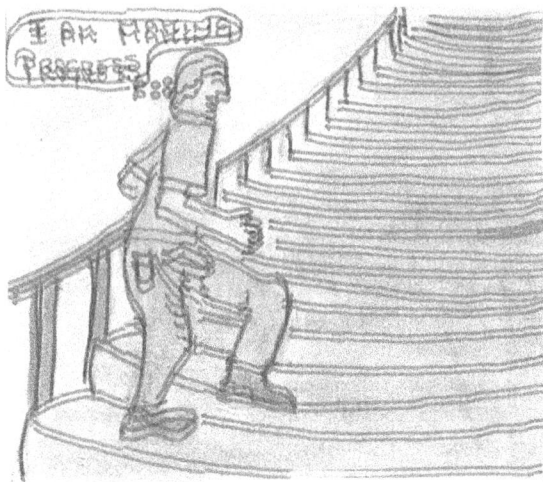

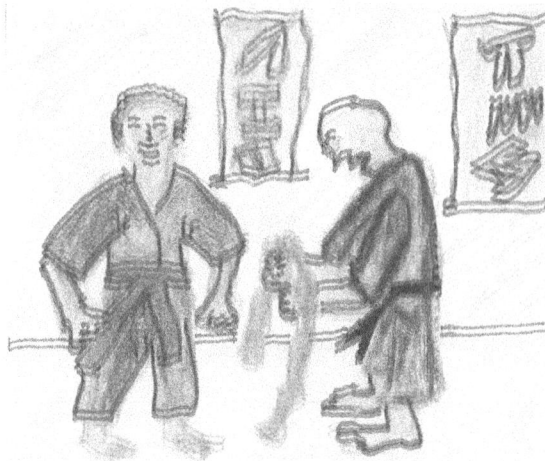

Break long-term goals down into short steps.	Once you feel comfortable, move onto your next short-term goal.

ACHIEVING LONG-TERM GOALS.

The prospect of taking on a long-term goal can often be so daunting that we usually prefer to put it off for a rainy day. Even when we are feeling well it is hard to contemplate, let alone when we are feeling depressed. If, however, we approach it by using a system of very short steps, or short-term goals, we can make the whole process a lot easier to cope with and far less daunting. If our long-term goal had been to run a marathon, then clearly there would have been no way that we could have just gone straight into a race without any training or preparation and that training would have to have involved gradually increasing the distance that we felt comfortable running. So our short-term goal would have been running various distances and once one distance was comfortably reached, then we would have our next short-term goal to be an even greater distance. This simple technique can be used to achieve any long-term goal and it is already very much a part of the way that w already live. For instance if you wanted to become a doctor, you would have to first get the right G.C.S.E.'s, then the right 'A' levels, then get into medical school, etc., etc. so it is common practice for all of us to use short-term goals in order to achieve our long-term goal.

Now do Exercise 31.

46

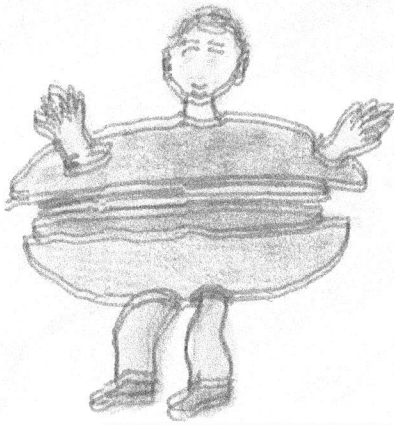

You are what you eat; "Hi, I'm Big Mac":		Aim to eat more fresh fruit salads and vegetables.

JUST WHAT IS A HEALTHY DIET?

There are literally hundreds of books out there about healthy diets, so if you feel that you want to go into a lot of details about it, I suggest that you buy one of them. Remember the saying "You are what you eat". Well there is a lot of truth in that; our bodies are made up of the food that we put into them, so clearly the better the food that we put into ourselves is, the healthier it is going to make us feel.

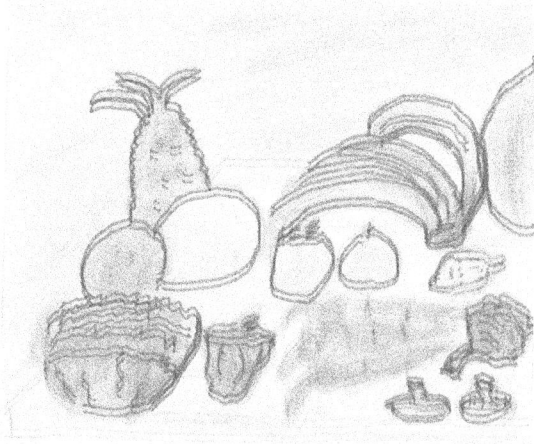

In general we need to eat lots of fresh fruit, salads and vegetables. We need to avoid fatty fried foods and processed foods, we need to cut down on red meat and we need to drink plenty of water. Most foods are fine in moderation and the occasional treat can help to raise our mood level, but if we can always try to keep to a varied diet that will give us all of the essential vitamins and minerals that we need, we will feel much healthier. Feeling good about our diet will go a long way to improving our feelings of self-worth.

Now do Exercise 32.

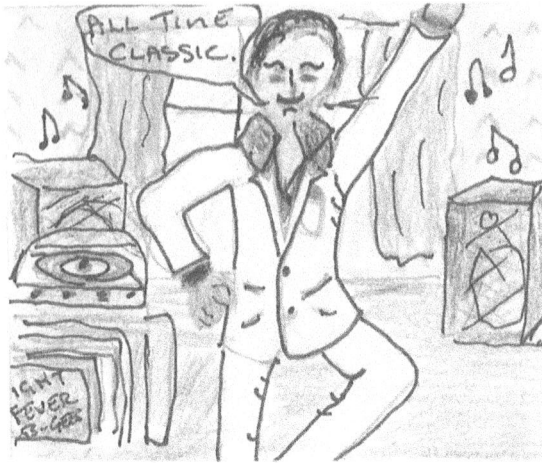

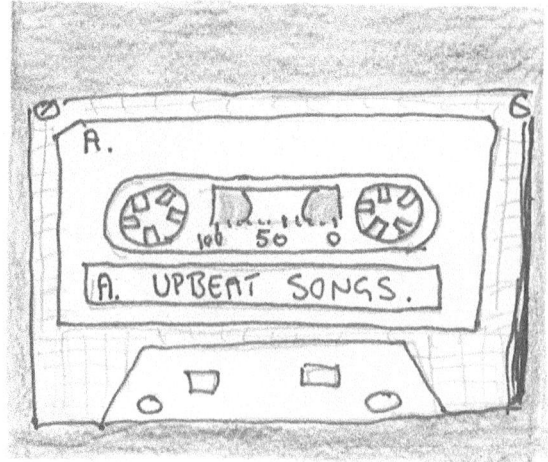

Use uplifting music to lift your spirits.		Make up a tape of your favourite upbeat songs.

CAN MUSIC HELP?

Music seems to have an incredible power over our emotions, with virtually an instantaneous effect. To ignore this incredible power over us would seem as ridiculous as ignoring the fact that we all feel uplifted by beautiful scenery. Music seems to be able to hit a raw nerve in us that nothing else ever seems to reach. If music has the power to completely change our mood, then surely we should be harnessing that power and using it to our own advantage. A lot of us give up listening to music when we are feeling depressed, or we only listen to sad slow mournful music.

What we really need to be listening to is as much upbeat adrenaline charged music as possible. Dance music can be particularly uplifting, look for songs that make you feel good about life and avoid songs that make you sit and dwell upon the meaning of things. Use music to help you, not to bring you down.

Now do Exercise 33.

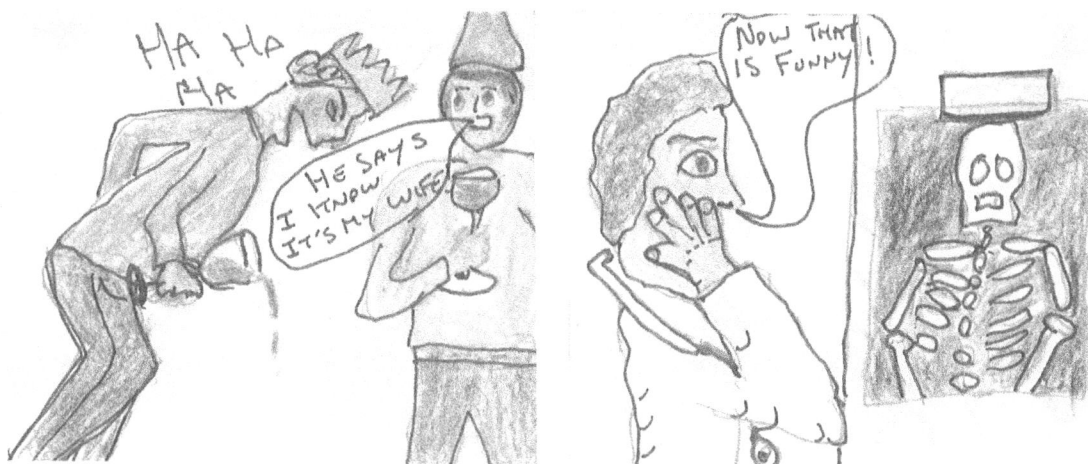

Having a good laugh is very good for you.		It can even stop terminal illness from progressing.

WHAT CAN LAUGHTER DO FOR ME WHEN I AM DEPRESSED?

One of the first things that we lose when we become depressed is our sense of humour. It can sometimes feel wrong or inappropriate to laugh when we are suffering from depression. This is a shame because when we can see the funny side of things, life becomes a lot more enjoyable. Being able to laugh is an essential part of feeling well and maintaining our well being.

It can also have a very positive knock-on effect throughout our entire bodies. Some people suffering from illnesses have been able to not only stop, but also reverse the onset of their disease by using laughter therapy. Laughter therapy involves gathering together all of the funny books that you have ever read all of the comedy films that you have enjoyed and all of the videos and tapes that you can find of your favourite comedians. Then set aside as much time as possible everyday to put them on so that you can have a good hearty laugh without feeling guilty. This should be a lot easier to do now that you know that it is an essential part of the recovery process.

Now do Exercise 34.

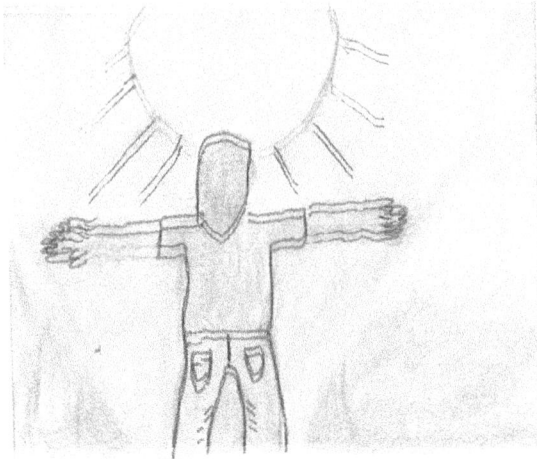

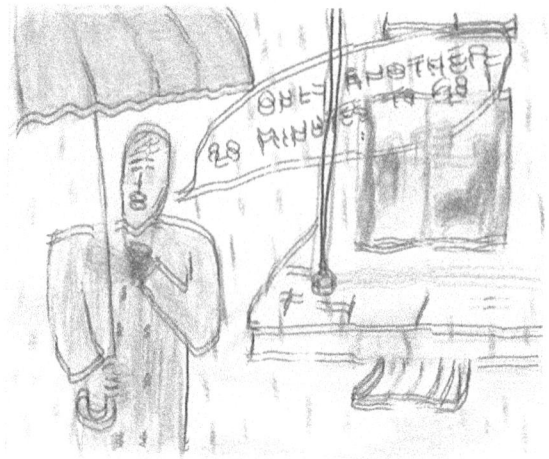

We need natural light everyday for nutrients and vitamins.		Get outside for at least thirty minutes every day.

GET SOME NATURAL LIGHT EVERY DAY.

During the summer months most of us tend to feel a lot better than we do in the winter months. This is because we are probably not exposing ourselves to enough natural full spectrum light, which provides us with the valuable vitamins and nutrients that we need. If we do not get at least thirty minute soft natural full spectrum light every day, then we can start to feel run down and fatigued. If these feelings persist they can lead to feelings of depression, or a similar condition referred to as SADS, (Seasonal Affective Disorder). Our bodies are not designed to be bombarded with things like neon lights, TV images, computer screens and interior shopping malls that have no natural light.

Make sure that you get outside for at least thirty minutes every day. Try and get into the habit of going for regular walks. You should soon feel less fatigued.

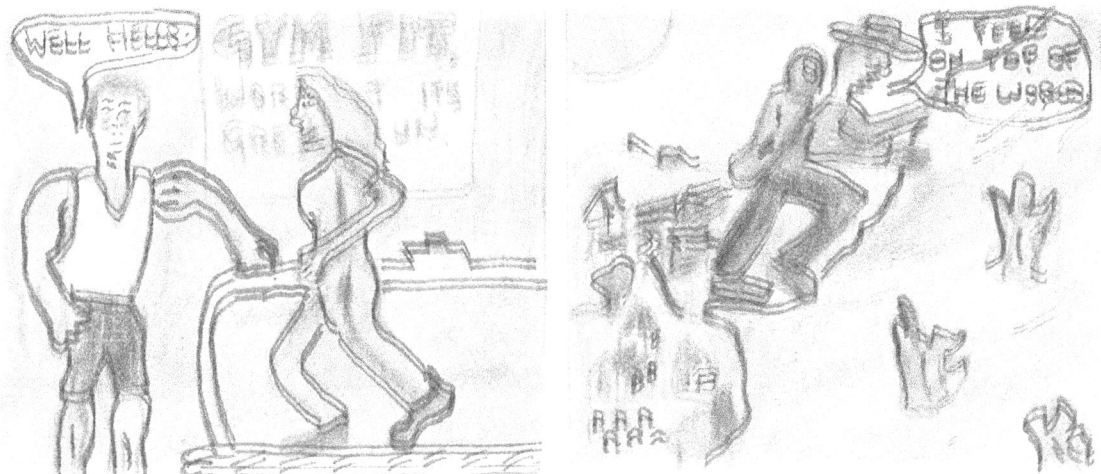

| It can improve your confidence and self-esteem. | | You will feel fitter, happier, and healthier. |

WHAT CAN EXERCISE DO FOR ME?

Exercise can do an awful lot for us whether we are depressed or not. Regular exercise is not only good for our bodies it is also good for our minds. Exercise releases the chemical endorphin into our blood stream. Nature's own natural feel-good drug. This gives us a natural high, which will help to lift our mood. Regular exercise also helps to maintain a regular routine (which is an essential part of keeping on course for recovery). It provides us with another opportunity to socialise and meet new people. It improves our physical well being, making us feel more comfortable about our own body image and our sense of self. It improves circulation and strengthens our hearts, which in turn promotes an improved sleeping pattern, allowing us to feel more relaxed and rested. Exercise gives us the opportunity to focus our minds away from our difficulties, as we have to put all of our concentration into the exercise; we learn to become focused. So exercise should help us with: concentration, self-esteem, confidence, assertiveness, relaxation, physical well-being, raising our mood level, stamina, endurance and fulfilment, along with helping to reinforce our belief and value system. Not bad for one activity!

Now do Exercise 35.

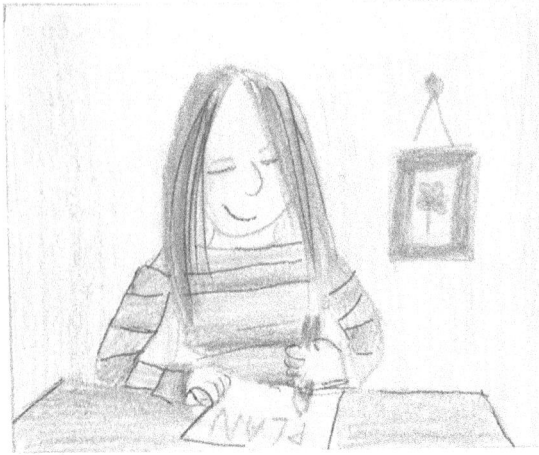

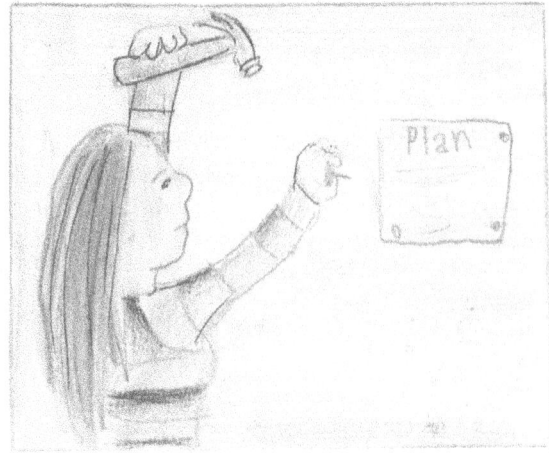

Convert the information that you have already gathered into a plan.	Stick your plan on your bedroom wall so that you can look at it every morning.

YOUR TREATMENT PLAN

Now that you have completed all of the exercises on depression, use the information that you have gathered to answer the following:

- I recognise that my depression is caused by …

- Things that are likely to make my depression worse are …

- I can make my life better by …

- I intend to improve my motivation by doing activities I want to do like …

- I intend to improve my mental fitness by …

- I intend to improve my inner harmony by using my values and beliefs to …

- My long-term goal is …

- I intend to improve my social life by …

- I promise to commit myself 100% to getting better by …

Now do Exercise 36

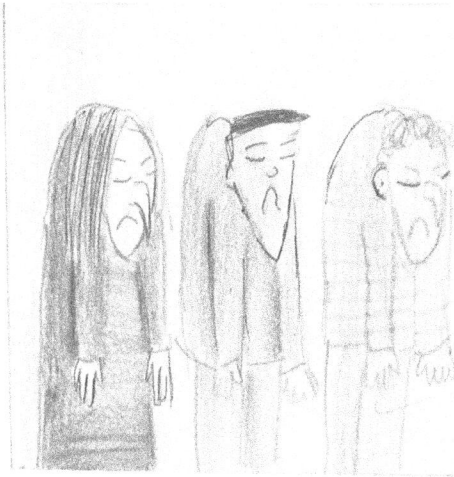

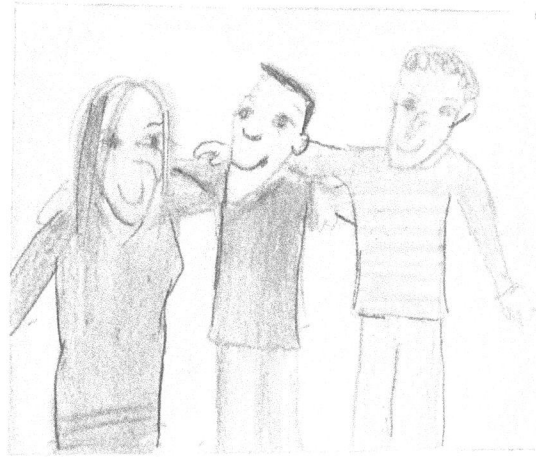

Don't let them make you feel useless.		Work with them to create a positive treatment plan, support them through it as much as you can.

WHAT CAN FAMILY AND FRIENDS DO TO HELP?

We can often be made to feel completely hopeless when confronted by somebody else's depression, particularly when it is a person that we deeply care for. We are all so wary about doing and saying the wrong thing, that very often we avoid the situation completely. Unfortunately, depressed people are very good at making us feel helpless, because they tend to reject any advice that we give them due to the fact that they are always looking for the negative and if you look hard enough you can find something negative in any situation.

This means that you have to be extra strong and positive when dealing with them, do not allow them to draw you into their negative thinking patterns, try to be optimistic at all times. Work with them to construct a treatment plan, perhaps you could do some activities with them or offer support in some way. Always show an interest in them. Praise them when they make an effort to change. Don't' be afraid to criticise them when they are destructive. Let them know that you are there for them and that you care about them, but keep some clear boundaries because it is vital that you also take good care of yourself.

DEPRESSION

DRUGS AND ALCOHOL

STRESS

ANXIETY

ANGER

LOW SELF-ESTEEM

POOR ASSERTIVENESS

Only a fool senses no fear,

A brave man is one who acknowledges his own fear,

But still manages to remain in control of his own destiny.

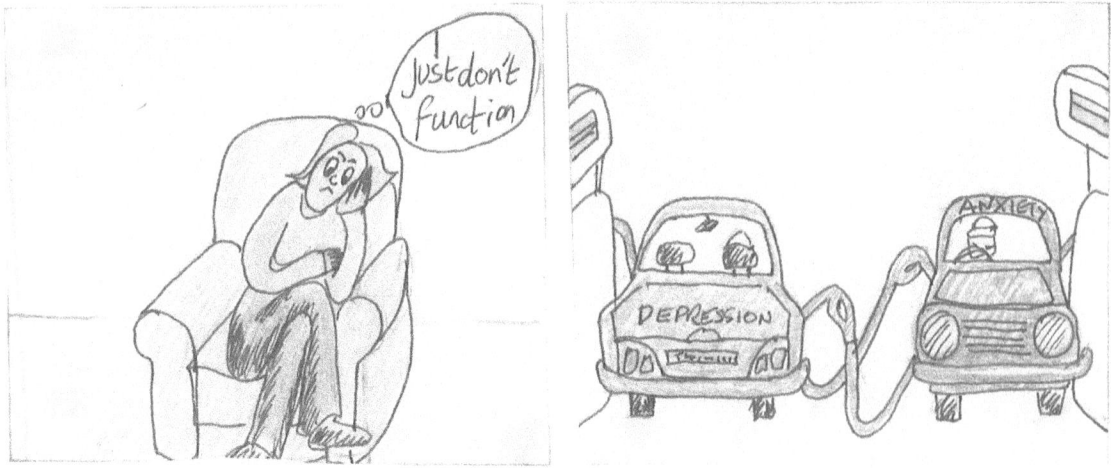

Most people who suffer from anxiety are also depressed.		Anxiety and depression tend to fuel each other.

THE LINK BETWEEN ANXIETY AND DEPRESSION.

About 80% of sufferers from either anxiety or depression are affected by both conditions together. So there is clearly a very strong link between the two. What tends to happen is that the two fuel each other; if you are feeling low and depressed you are going to see everything from a worse case scenario perspective, which means that you will expect bad things to happen to you, so you are highly likely to become anxious. You will also have ongoing concerns about yourself and your future, which are bound to raise your level of anxiety.

If you are suffering from anxiety, you are likely to get fed up and despondent with the constant effort that is required to do anything and you may reach a point when you start to withdraw from society. This can lead to low mood helplessness and depression.

Anxiety is a natural response to danger.		Unfortunately it does not help us to deal with modern day problems.

WHAT EXACTLY IS ANXIETY?

The word anxiety is used a lot by all of us, but what does it actually mean? Anxiety is a natural response to danger, it is not something that we can easily remove, nor should we ever want to, as it is vital for our own survival.

Anxiety works by preparing our bodies for immediate action so that we can cope with dangerous situations. This is sometimes referred to as the "fight or flight response", because we are quite literally preparing to either fight or run away.

Of course that is all very well if we are faced with a tiger, it becomes a very useful response. But in today's modern world our fears tend to be more complex, such as redundancy, relationship difficulties, debts, exam results, etc. (The list is endless). These are problems that we cannot run away from or fight with our fists, and so the anxiety response is of no use whatsoever to us. Yet it still happens and when it does our bodies and minds become very confused, because we do not understand how or why these awful feelings are happening to us and we do not know how to deal with them.

Now look at Exercise 37 on Anxiety at the back of the book.

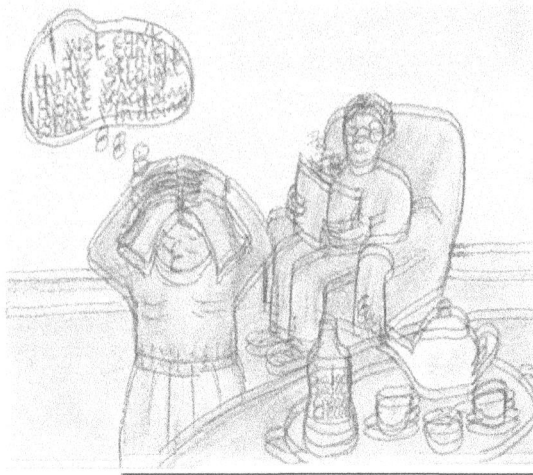

Anxiety has a profound effect upon the way that we think:		Anxiety also affects our behaviour.

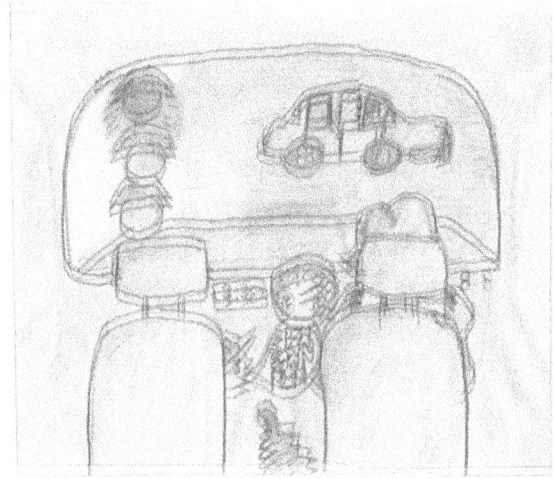

ANXIETY AFFECTS US PHYSICALLY, PSYCHOLOGICALLY AND BEHAVIOURLY:

Although most of us tend to regard anxiety as a purely physical response we need to be aware that it also has a strong psychological component to it as well as a behavioural one:

Our bodies need to be told that there is a danger in order to initiate a physical response in the first place and it is our minds that provide our bodies with that message. Often though, our minds perceive things incorrectly; this could be because we are feeling depressed, confused, vulnerable, or insecure. So we start to question our own mind's ability to correctly identify danger, making us feel even more insecure and vulnerable. Eventually the only trigger that we need to initiate an anxiety attack is our own fear of anxiety. This can lead to us using avoidance behaviour, which will have the effect of stopping us from going out for fear of having an anxiety attack. Or we will run away from places or people that we consider to be too anxiety provoking. This behaviour eventually becomes more disabling than the anxiety itself.

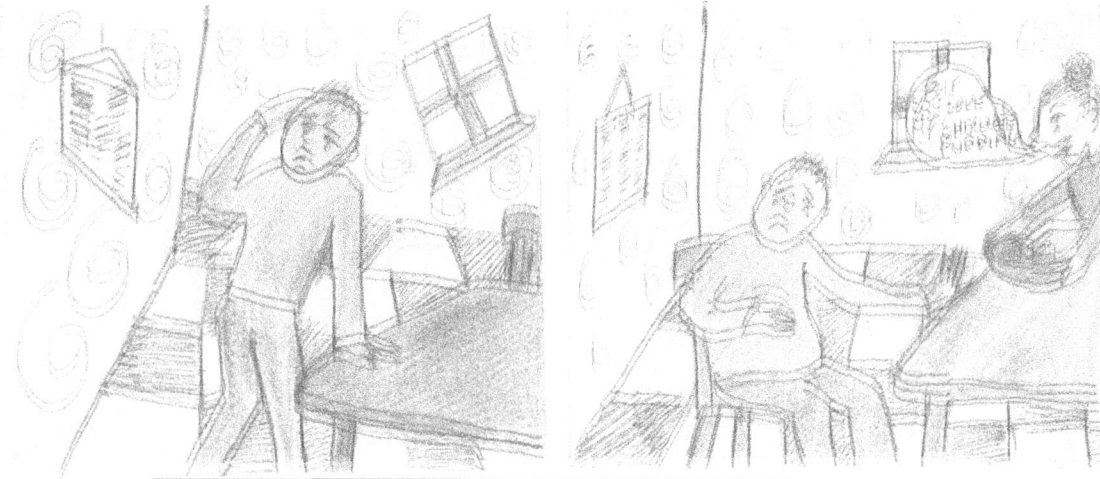

We can feel dizzy due to an increased level of blood flow.	Our stomach shuts down as we will not be eating in an emergency.

THE PHYSICAL EFFECTS OF ANXIETY.

As our bodies prepare to either fight or run away, adrenaline is secreted and our bodies start to adapt in order to be able to deal with the immediate crisis as effectively as possible.

Blood is taken away from some of our organs, whose functions will not be required when it comes to dealing with the present crisis, organs such as the stomach, because we certainly won't be stopping for a bite to eat in the middle of a threatening situation! Extra blood is then pumped to all of the organs that we may need to use, such as the brain for quick thinking, the ears and eyes for increased awareness, the muscles for extra strength. All other physical symptoms that we experience come about as a direct result of these changes. Symptoms such as increased sweating, blurred vision, bowel problems, shaking, nausea migraines and chest pains, breathing difficulties and muscle cramps.

Now do Exercise 38.

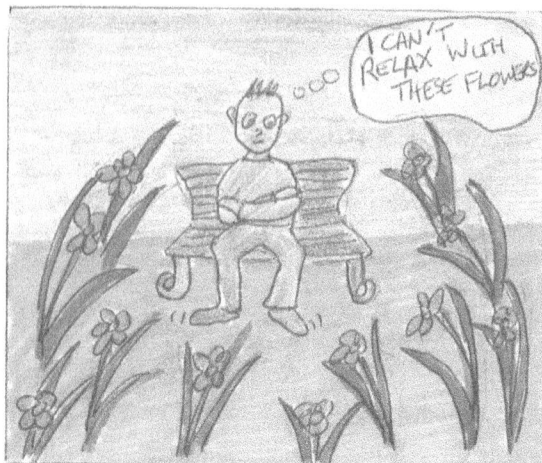

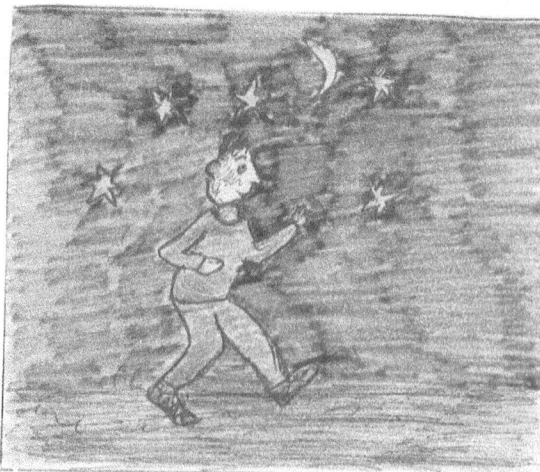

Our bodies react to the information that we give them.	We can become afraid of the physical changes that happen.

OUR PERCEPTION CAN PUT US IN A SPIN.

What we perceive as something dreadful happening to our bodies is in fact the opposite, our bodies are trying to work properly in response to the information that we have just supplied them with. It is therefore the information that we are sending that is the problem not the response.

When we tell our bodies that we are faced with a dangerous situation, our bodies respond by preparing to deal with it. The trouble is that it is often the changes taking place in our bodies that we become aware of first. So we perceive it as a purely physical malfunction. This will then start us off on a spiral of worry. Am I going to have a heart attack? What is wrong with me? The more we worry the more our bodies prepare for imminent danger by increasing their physical responses.

Now do Exercise 39.

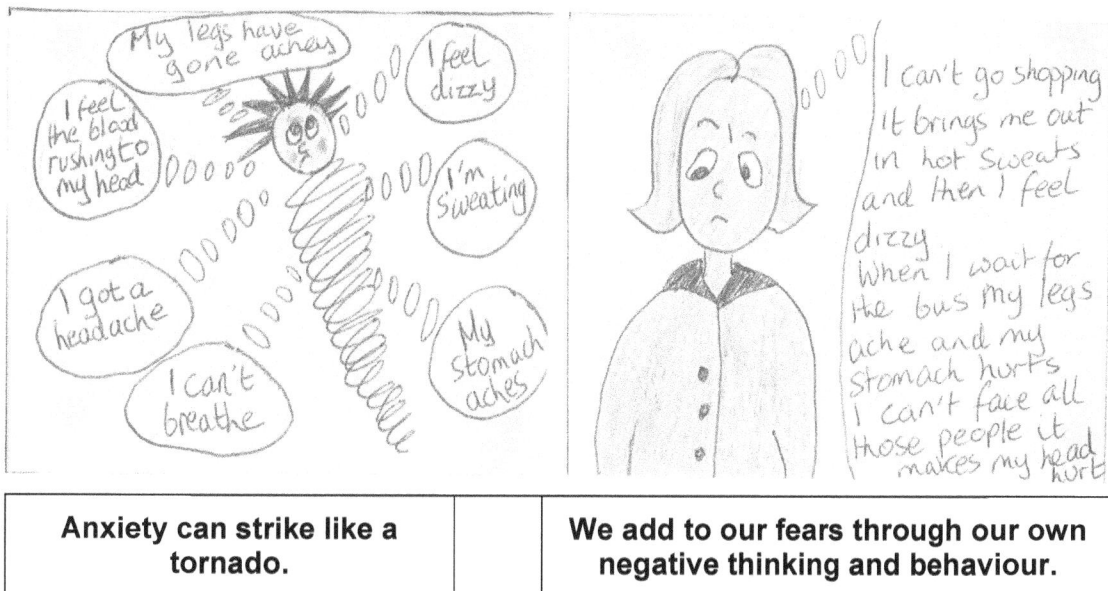

Anxiety can strike like a tornado.	We add to our fears through our own negative thinking and behaviour.

HOW ANXIETY ATTACKS US.

Anxiety always attacks us like a tornado because once something has triggered it off we keep adding to it with our own negative spiral of thinking and behaving. Let's see how it works.

- Something triggers us to think "I hope I am not going to get anxious again because I can't cope with that!"

- We then check for any physical signs of anxiety, which will be starting to occur because we have just frightened ourselves.

- We become afraid of the inevitable anxiety attack. We blame it all on our environment so we make an effort to escape and run away, thereby making us feel even more vulnerable.

- Our minds are now fully focused upon how dreadful we are feeling.

- We tell ourselves that we cannot cope, making us more afraid.

- This cycle goes on and on fuelling itself like a tornado.

Now do Exercise 55.

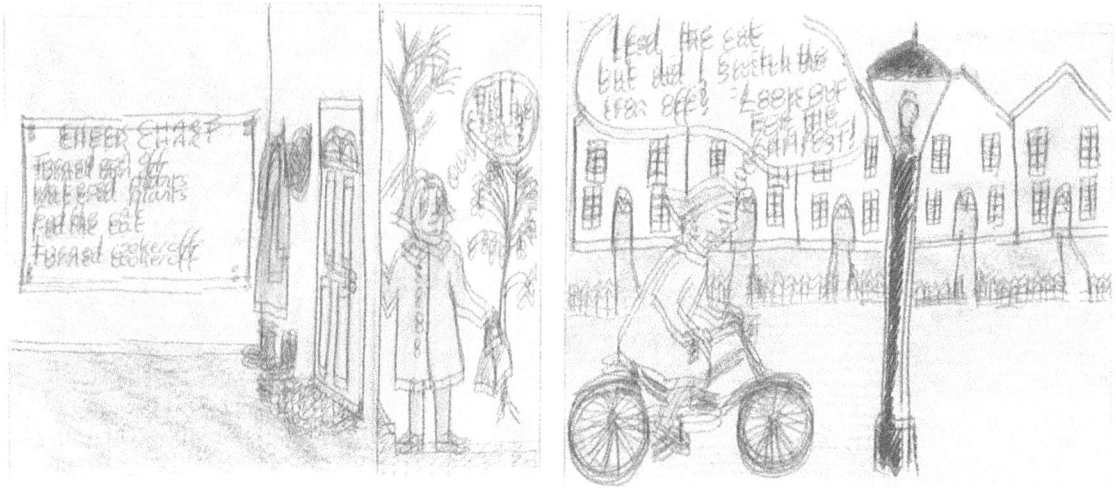

We can start to check things over and over again.		It should help you to make the most out of your life.

ASSOCIATED DIFFICULTIES.

Some people with anxiety go on to develop a condition called obsessive-compulsive disorder. This is very disabling for the sufferer because they start to develop a series of rituals or repetitive habits that must be performed regularly in order to keep the anxiety at bay. It is very similar to the superstitions that most of us used as children; such as "If I don't step on any cracks in the pavement, I'll get that toy car for my birthday".

Most compulsions take the form of checking behaviours, such as turning the light switch off ten times, or checking that the cooker is turned off a set number of times before going to bed.

These compulsions can make it virtually impossible to lead a normal life, as they start to affect and control everything that we do. The only way that we can conquer these compulsions is to learn how to deal effectively with our anxiety, so that we no longer fear it.

Now do Exercise 41.

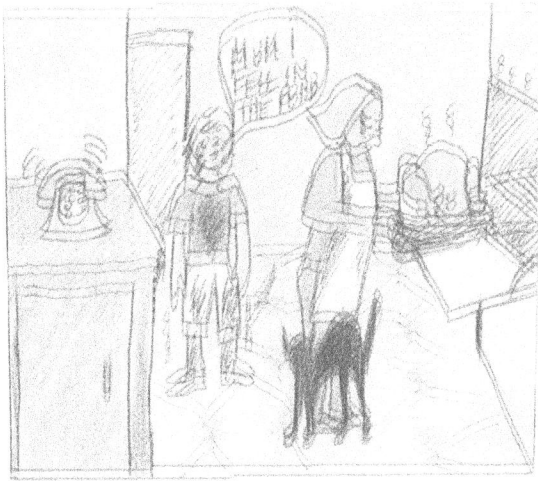

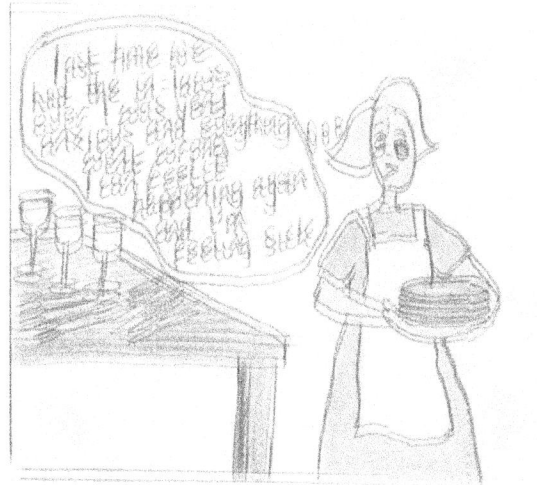

| Many different things can trigger off our anxiety. | | Ironically the fear of anxiety itself can become a major trigger. |

TRIGGERS.

A trigger is anything at all that can initiate an anxiety response in us. It could be travelling on public transport, going into a busy shop, going to the cinema, large groups of people, dogs or even leaving the safety of our own home. Absolutely anything can act as a trigger if it is capable of managing to frighten us.

The ironic thing is that it is often the fear of having an anxiety attack itself that can act as a trigger. Sometimes the trigger can be so well buried into our subconscious that we can be completely unaware of it until we start to analyse our anxiety patterns in some detail.

Once we identify and analyse why these triggers are having such an effect upon us, we can reduce their impact on us by coming up with some alternative view points that have more positive outcomes.

Now do Exercise 42.

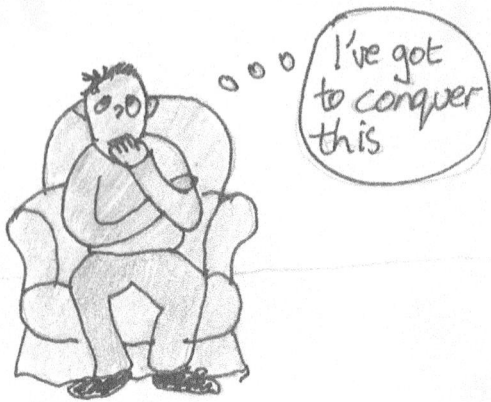

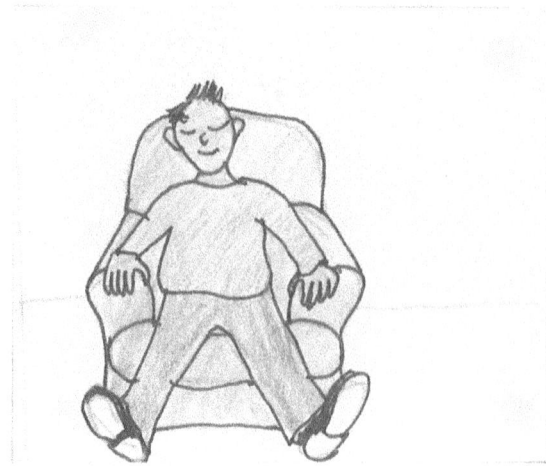

There are four main approaches to conquering anxiety.	Learn how to relax property.

HOW DO WE CONQUER ANXIETY?

There are four main approaches that we can take when it comes to conquering anxiety. They will all take a lot of time and patience, but they do all work eventually. The first approach is RELAXATION. When we suffer from anxiety attacks we also know exactly how it feels to recover from them. When we recover from an anxiety attack, one of the first things that we notice is just how much more relaxed we feel. Being in a relaxed state is the complete opposite of being in an anxious state; this is why we need to learn how to relax as quickly and effectively as possible whenever we are faced with an anxiety-provoking situation.

In order to be able to achieve quick and effective relaxation we need to practise our relaxation techniques on a regular basis. If we can learn to counteract the physical effects of anxiety as soon as they happen to us, then we will be able to stop anxiety attacks in their tracks.

Now do Exercise 43.

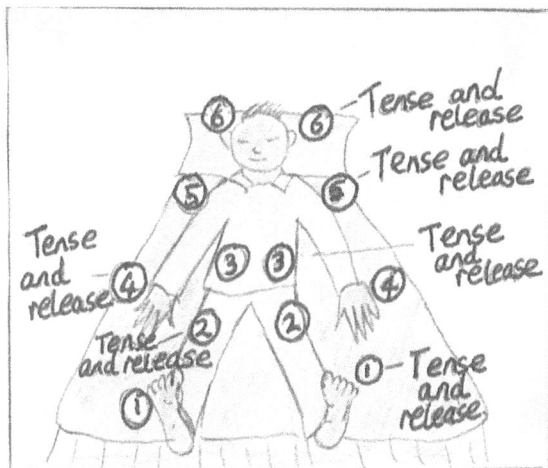

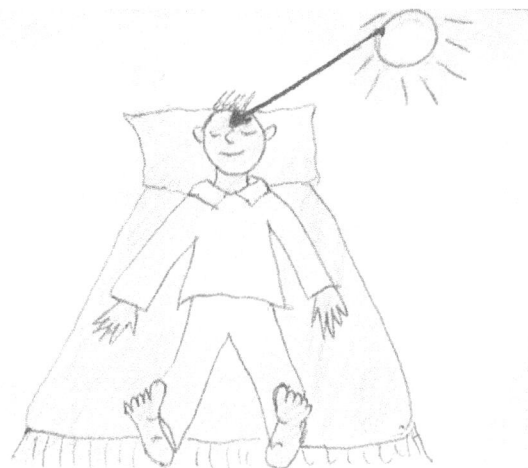

Lie down, tense and release muscles one at a time.		Try to focus upon a healing white light.

RELAXATION EXERCISE.

- Find a quiet room where you are unlikely to be disturbed.

- Remove your shoes and any tight clothing.

- Lie flat on a bed or on the floor and close your eyes.

- Starting with your toes, practise tensing up your muscles, one at a time, holding the tension for about 15 seconds, before releasing it.

- As you release focus upon your muscles becoming heavy and sinking into the floor.

- Use this technique for all of your muscles working your way up.

- Concentrate on your ears, imagine sound being pushed out rather than taken in.

- Now tense up each eye one at a time and then let them relax while you focus upon the space between them, your middle eye.

- Focus on a beam of clear white light entering your body through your middle eye; this is a healing light that brings goodness into your body.

- Try to hold onto this image, letting nothing else enter your mind for as long as possible.

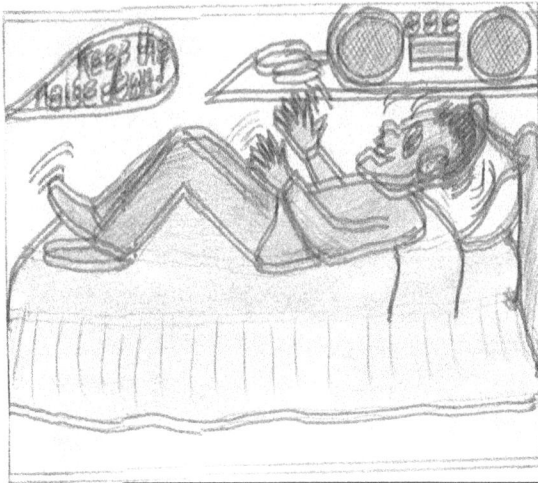

Relax to a soothing piece of music.		Have a good laugh with some friends.

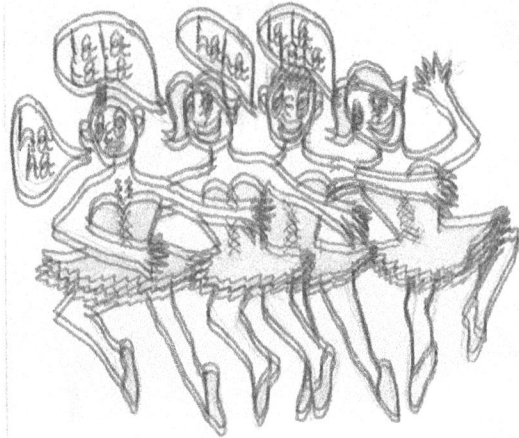

ADOPT A MORE RELAXED LIFESTYLE.

If things are getting on top of us to such an extent that we are continually feeling anxious, then we clearly need to adopt a more light-hearted approach to our lives. Getting anxious and worked up about things does not help us to deal with them any better, whereas a more relaxed approach to things can often work wonders.

We need to learn how to switch off and relax to a soothing piece of music. We need to learn to appreciate the natural beauty all around us. We need to spend some time enjoying ourselves and doing some of the things that we want to do, like having a good laugh with some friends. If we are more relaxed our ability to rationally problem solve improves drastically and so therefore does our ability to deal with anxiety.

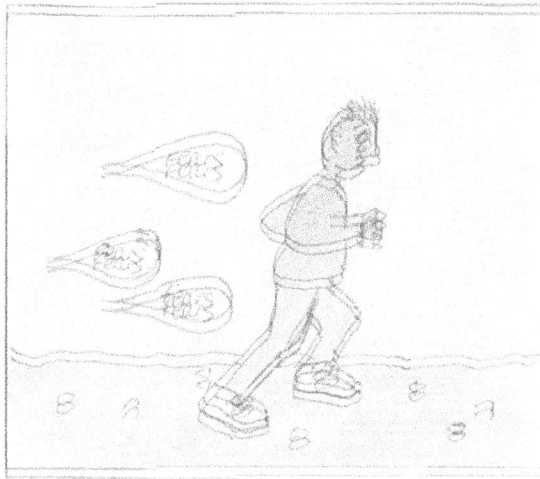

| Step running away from your fears. | | It is time to take control of your own fears. |

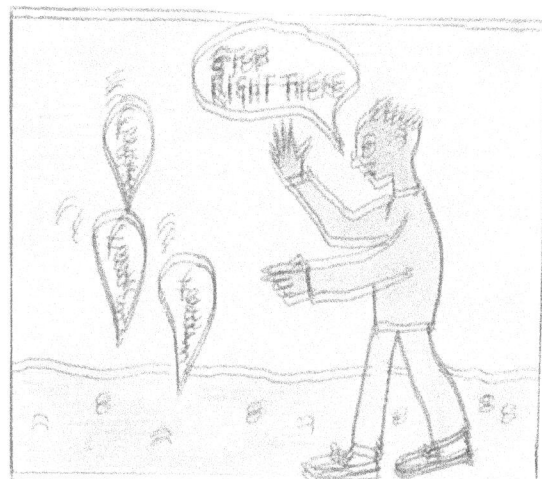

WE NEED TO CHANGE OUR BEHAVIOUR.

We cannot allow ourselves to be controlled and debilitated by anxiety, we have to tell ourselves that we are going to fight back and regain control. Every time that we give in to the urge to run away from a shop, or avoid the man coming the other way, we are fuelling our anxiety making it stronger and stronger.

Anxiety knows no boundaries and unless we learn how to fight it, it will go on controlling us more and more. Unfortunately nobody else can fight it for us. Once we start to gain some control over our anxiety, we reverse the negative cycle into a positive one. Every time that we manage to prevent an anxiety attack from occurring, we equip ourselves better to cope with the next possible attack.

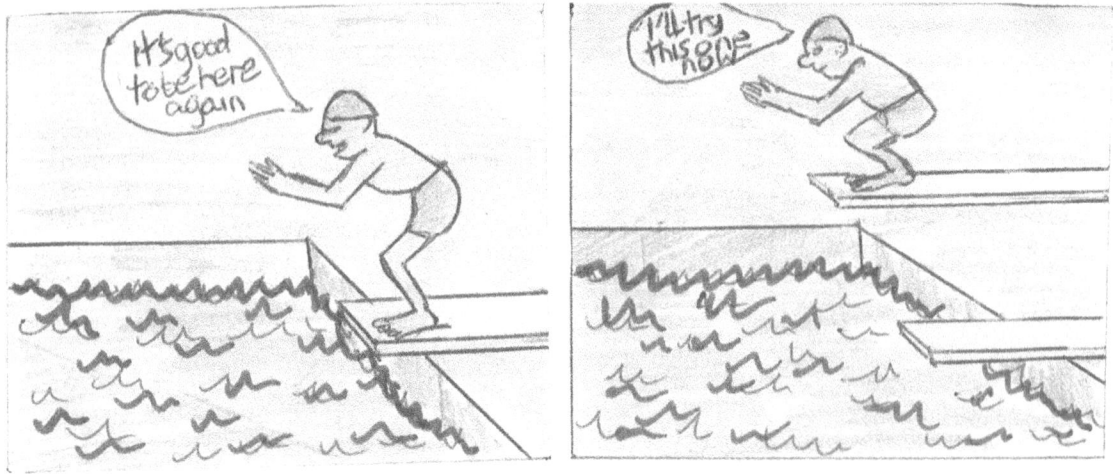

Get used to going to a place.		Gradually increase what you can do.

WE CAN TAKE SOME POSITIVE STEPS.

Chose one of the least threatening places on your list of anxiety provoking situations, making sure that it is somewhere that you would really like to be able to go. You can now use that as your goal to work towards achieving. All that you have to do next is to break that goal down into lots of smaller goals or steps. Here is an example using returning to diving at the local swimming pool as our long-term goal.

- Walk to the swimming pool with a friend.

- Walk to the swimming pool with a friend and go in for a cup of tea.

- Walk to the swimming pool on your own.

- Walk to the swimming pool on your own and buy a cup of tea.

- Go swimming with your friend for 20 minutes.

- Go swimming while your friend has a cup of tea for 15 minutes.

- Go swimming on your own for 15 minutes.

- Go swimming on your own for 25 minutes.

- Go swimming and use the diving board.

- Reward yourself for achieving your long-term goal.

Now do Exercise 44.

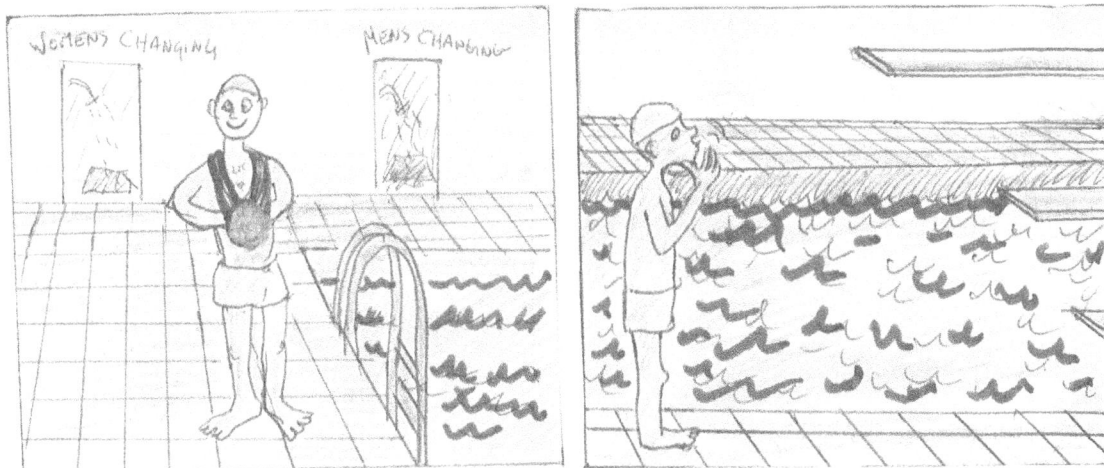

Give yourself a reward for your achievements to date.		Plan your next goal.

WE NEED TO BE ABLE TO REWARD OURSELVES.

The good thing about the step approach is that it allows us to spend as much or as little time as we need to cover each step. Then only when we feel ready do we decide to try and move onto the next step. So if for any reason we struggle, we know that we only need to return to the previous step and not the very beginning.

When we achieve a goal we need to get into the habit of praising and rewarding ourselves, after all we know that it is not easy otherwise we wouldn't be doing it in the first place!

So we need to buy ourselves a small gift or treat ourselves to something special. We need to learn to value ourselves and the progress that we are making. We should enjoy the newfound freedom that we have helped to create as we finally start to control our anxiety rather than letting it control us.

Now do Exercise 45.

Learn to recognise your own negative thoughts.	Try using an elastic band to snap yourself out of negative thinking.

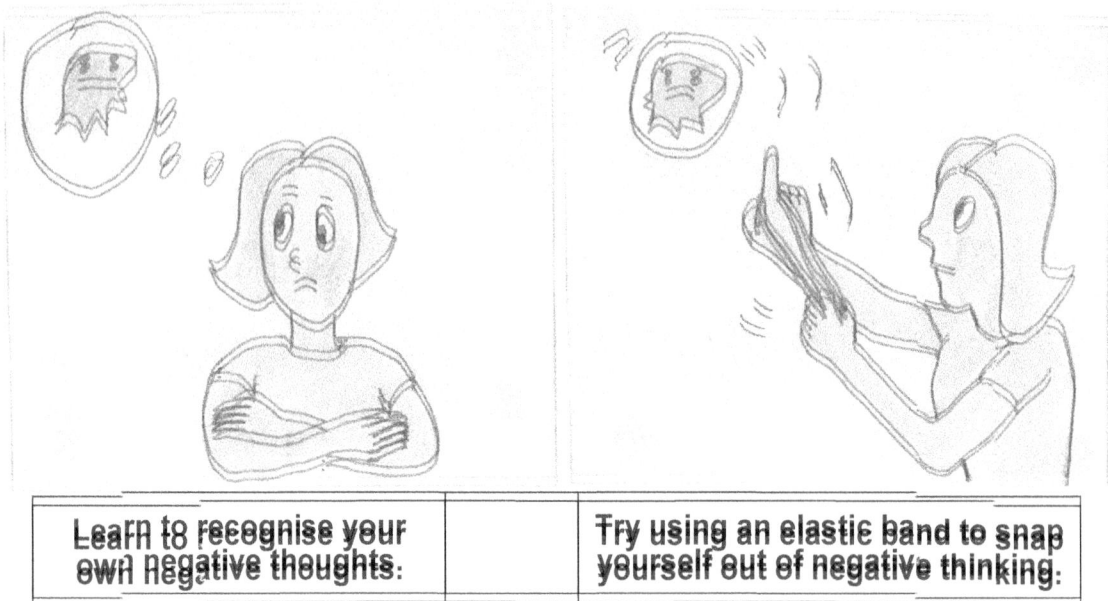

WE NEED TO PREVENT NEGATIVE THINKING.

There are a lot of books that we could read, which could tell us about all the various classifications of thinking errors that there are but do we really need to know them? The fact is that if we are prone to anxiety and depression, we are also prone to negative thinking. This could be down to our genetic make-up or our life experiences to date.

Either way we have to accept that negative thinking is a very destructive mechanism, which does tend to work as a self-fulfilling prophecy. Negative thinking keeps us locked into a cycle of anxiety that we need to learn to break.

The first step that we need to learn is how to recognise when we are having negative thoughts. We need to get used to constantly double-checking them. Some people wear an elastic band around their wrist so that they can twang themselves every time that they think negatively, this gives them a chance to consider some more positive alternatives.

Now do Exercise 46.

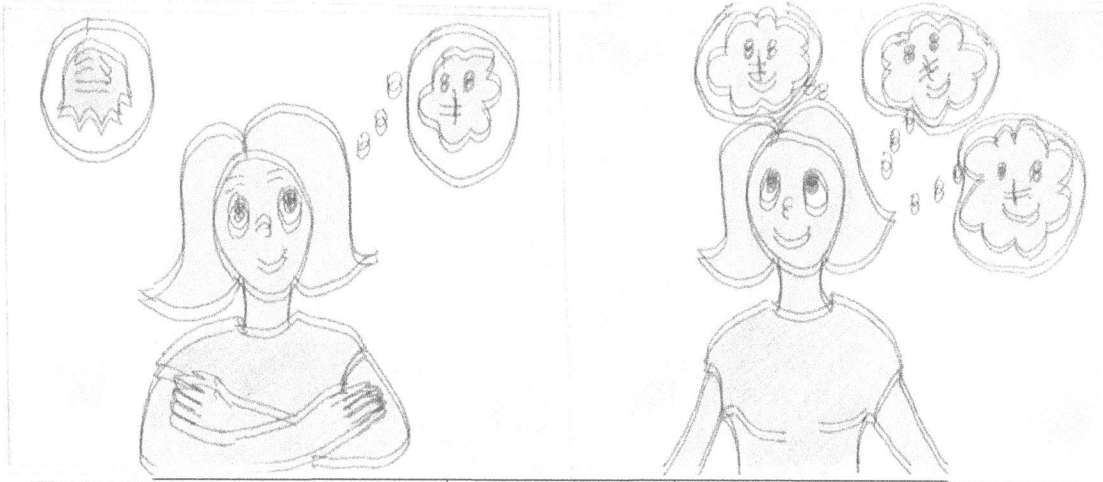

Counteract negative thoughts.		Keep practicing until it comes naturally.

COUNTERACT THOSE NEGATIVE THOUGHTS WITH POSITIVE ONES.

Every time that you have a negative thought about anything, you need to come back immediately with a positive thought about the same thing.

Example 1.

Negative Thought = *This is an awful rundown looking town.*

Positive Thought = *It does have some very good facilities such as a modern library and a large swimming pool.*

Example 2.

Negative Thought = *That man looks dreadful in those awful clothes.*

Positive Thought = *It's good to see people express themselves through fashion, it makes the world a more interesting place.*

These positive challenges can be applied to absolutely anything, all we have to do is keep practising until it becomes second nature.

Now do Exercise 47

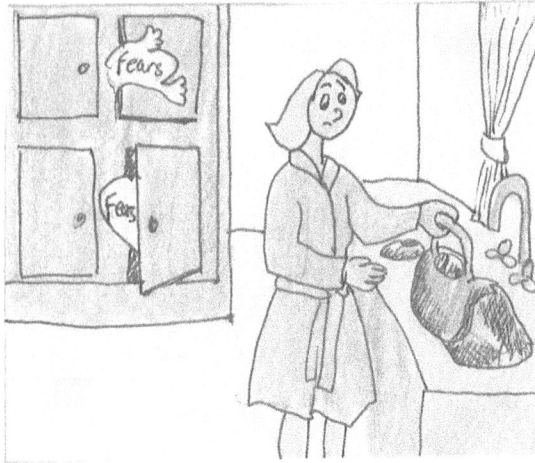

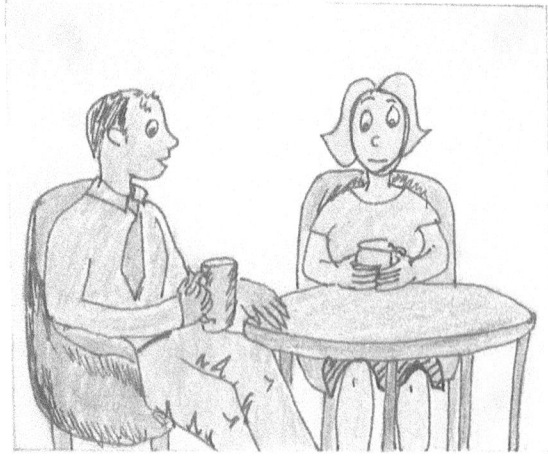

Do you have hidden fears?		Explore the beliefs behind the fears with a counsellor.

FACE YOUR FEARS HEAD ON.

In some cases it is possible for us to stop the anxiety altogether, just by developing a deeper insight and awareness into our own fears. Although possible, this can sometimes prove to be a very difficult task to achieve on our own, so it can often be very beneficial for us to seek out the services of an experienced counsellor.

The technique most often used involves stripping our irrational beliefs down to the bare bones, so that we can understand where they originally cam from and just how illogical they really are. We can then hopefully change the dysfunctional belief and eradicate the fear that has been triggering our anxiety.

If we want to try this technique ourselves, all that we have to do is identify a belief that we currently hold then keep asking ourselves why? If we answer the question honestly each time until we can go not further, we will eventually be able to identify our own core dysfunctional belief. Once we know and understand this belief, we can choose whether or not we want to change it.

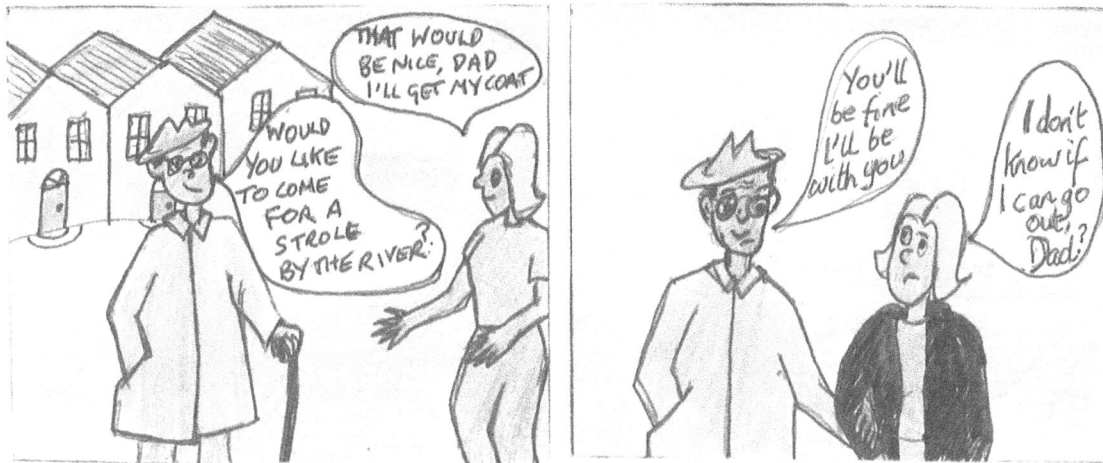

Carry out activities together.		Always be strong, positive and patient.

WHAT CAN YOUR FAMILY AND FRIENDS DO TO HELP?

Most people will choose to either avoid you or try to do everything for you when you are suffering from anxiety. Unfortunately, neither of these approaches are very helpful.

The best way that anybody can help a sufferer of anxiety is to adopt and approach of encouragement and joint working, in other words encourage the sufferer to do tasks with you. Don't be tempted to do their shopping for them, even though it seems like a very helpful and logical approach; in the long run it will make them more dependent and anxious.

Instead you need to encourage them to do things with you, so offer to go shopping with them. Offer to do domestic chores together. Support them with the treatment regimes in this book; encourage them to attend leisure pursuits with you. Be there for them as an optimistic friend and always be strong and positive when in their company.

DEPRESSION

DRUGS AND ALCOHOL

ANXIETY

STRESS

ANGER

LOW SELF-ESTEEM

POOR ASSERTIVENESS

A man who has forgotten how to enjoy and appreciate the good things in life,

Will soon only become familiar with the sad and bad things in life.

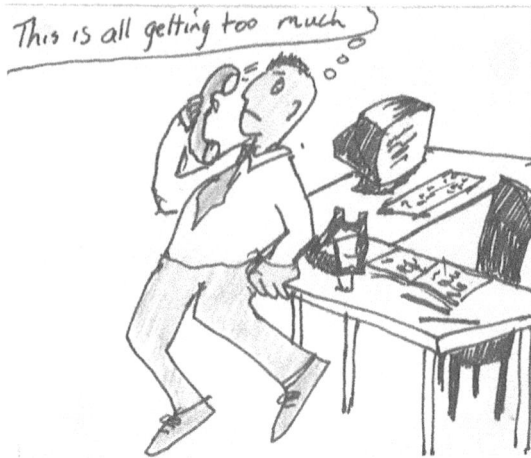

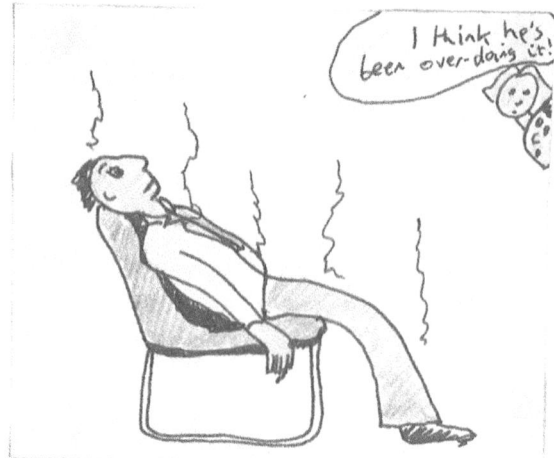

| Stress is a prolonged feeling of arousal maintained by ongoing difficulties. | Our bodies are not designed to cope with it, so they burn out. |

HOW DOES STRESS DIFFER FROM ANXIETY?

Stress and anxiety tend to share a lot of symptoms, so just what is the difference between the two of them? Anxiety tends to be a quick, severe, overwhelming attack, whereas stress is a less severe, but more continuous, constant level of high arousal. The trouble for us is that our bodies are not designed to maintain this level of functioning for long periods of time. So if the stressors persist without us mastering ways of decreasing their threat, we can reach a state known as "burn out". This is when we reach a state of total physical and mental exhaustion.

Now do Exercise 48.

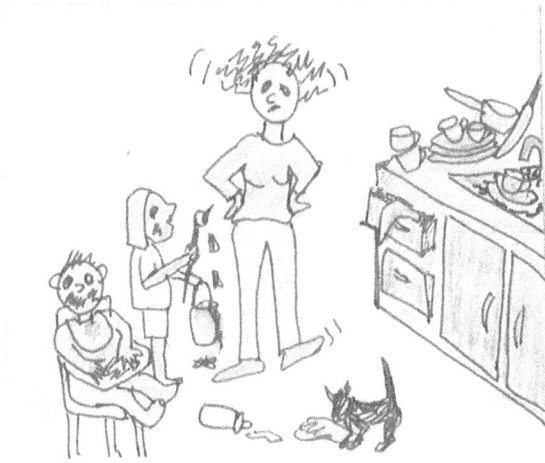

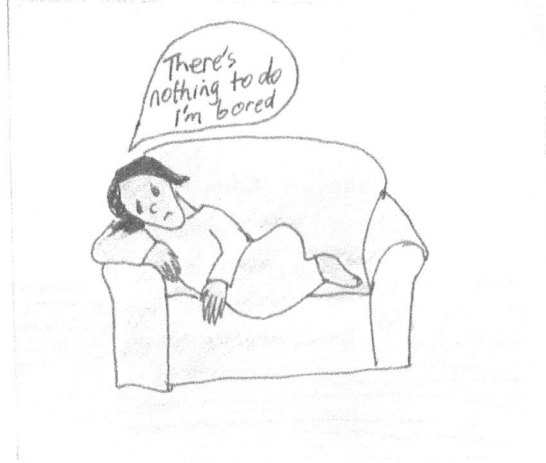

| When we feel unable to deal with things our stress level rises. | We can also feel stressed if we are bored and our minds are not stimulated. |

WHAT IS STRESS?

Stress is a word that we use a lot to describe how we sometimes feel but what does it actually mean? In it's simplest form, stress is the state that we experience when the demands that are made upon us cannot be counter-balanced by our ability to deal with them.

It is how we see those demands and how capable we feel about dealing with them that will ultimately decide whether we feel completely overwhelmed on one extreme or bored stiff on the other.

There is a middle ground or course, when the demands made upon us are stimulating and our coping resources feel perfectly able to deal with them. This is a satisfying and rewarding situation to be in because we are neither bored nor stressed; we are functioning at an appropriate level, which leaves us feeling content.

Now do Exercise 49.

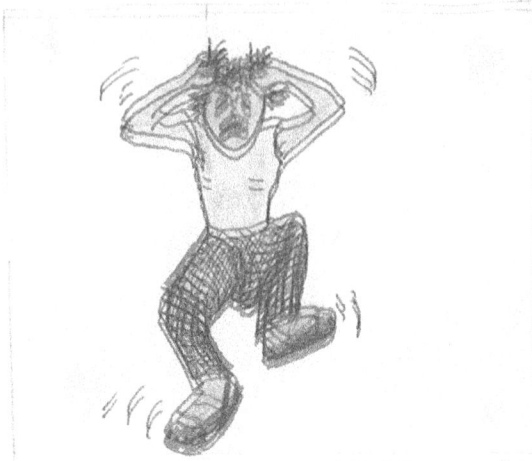

We can become highly-strung and over-emotional.		Our minds tell our body that it is not coping so our body reacts.

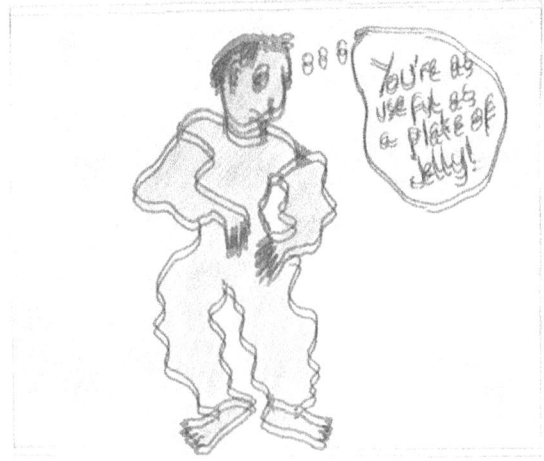

HOW DOES STRESS AFFECT US?

The symptoms of stress can vary greatly from person to person. In the early stages most people will feel very emotional, often becoming tearful or short-tempered, they can become easily agitated, muscles become tense, they have difficulty relaxing, they may start to feel physically and mentally exhausted.

These symptoms occur because the mind tells the body that it is not coping and so the body reacts in the only way that it knows how, by secreting more adrenaline, and preparing the body for action. Unfortunately this response is not suitable or helpful when it comes to dealing with a lot of today's sorts of problems. So the effect upon our bodies only serves to make us feel worse, we become angry with ourselves and we struggle even more to cope with the situation.

Now do Exercise 50.

78

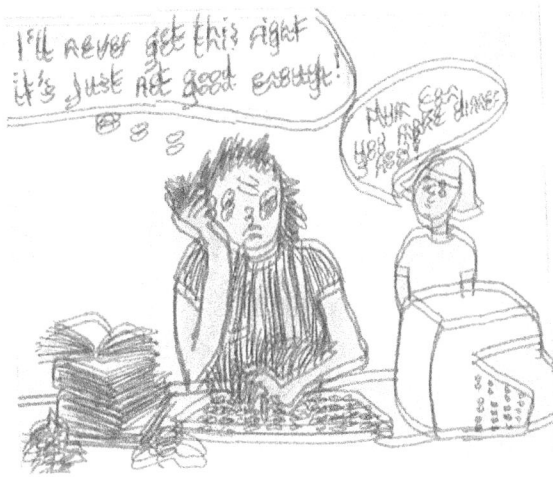

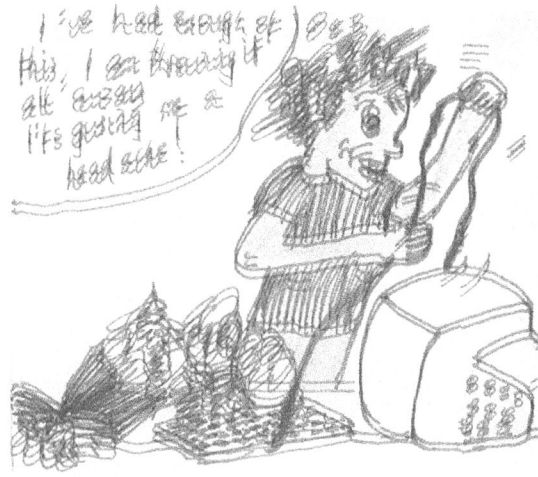

Stress tends to affect people who are demanding upon themselves.	Stress can be the cause of many behavioural and physical problems.

WHAT CAN STRESS DO TO YOU?

The majority of people who suffer from stress tend to be very demanding upon themselves; they believe that they should be able to cope with any situation. So when they find themselves unable to function at all due to "burn out", they become completely devastated and depressed.

Long-term stress can also cause muscle and bone deformities, due to excessive prolonged tension. It can cause heart problems due to increased prolonged blood pressure. It can also be the cause of migraines, allergies, blurred vision and poor digestion.

Behaviourally stress can make you short-fused, nervous, agitated, anti-social and reclusive. So all in all anyone suffering from stress stands a very high chance of developing depression.

Now do Exercise 51:

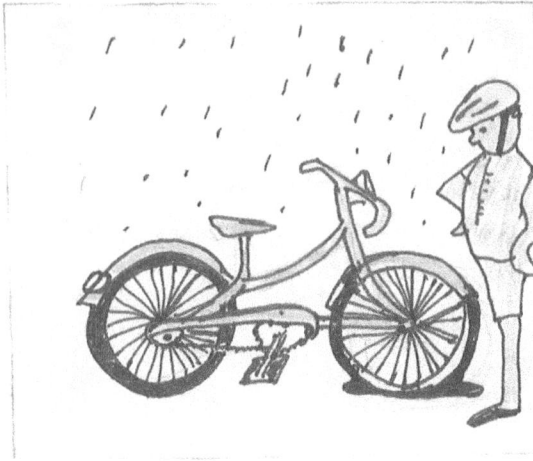

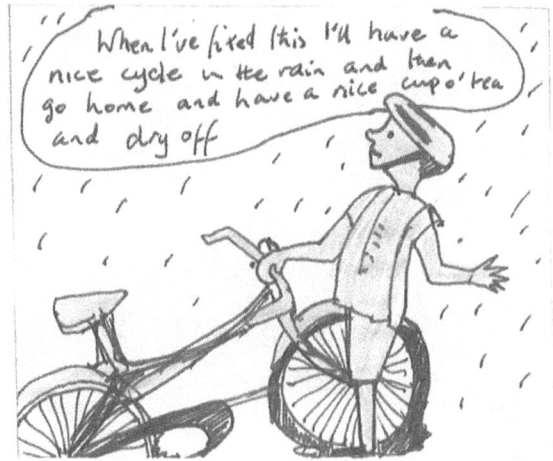

Anything at all can cause you to suffer from stress.		It is how we perceive it that determines how stressed we are going to feel.

THE CAUSES OF STRESS.

Absolutely anything can be the cause of stress. We are all different in the way that we view things; one man's pleasure is another man's nightmare. The real difference comes in the way that we perceive the situation. Two people can be faced with exactly the same difficulty, but if they perceive it differently their responses will be very different.

With an increase in stress levels comes a decrease in coping skills. Our negative perceptions continue to increase, making every dilemma more and more threatening and difficult to deal with. Stress can therefore be said to have a self-perpetuating effect.

Now do Exercise 52.

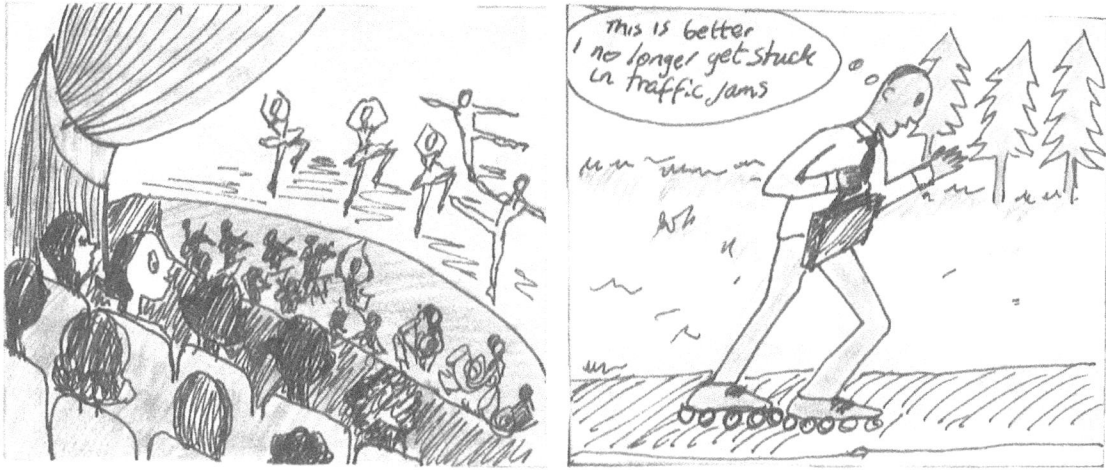

It can be good to get away from our stress.		We need to learn new skills so that things seem less threatening.

SOME WAYS THAT WE CAN CONQUER STRESS.

One of the best ways to conquer stress is to remove ourselves from the stressor and avoid the situation altogether. Unfortunately it is not always possible to be able to take this approach because many stressful things cannot be avoided. For instance, work can be a major stressor in a lot of people's lives, but it is not always easy for us to change our occupations and if we did give up our jobs we would be exposing ourselves to another major stressor, lack of money! So sometimes we have to put up with some stressors in order to avoid others. Another way that we can avoid stress is by learning to adapt to the demands made upon us. If we can learn to plan ahead and prepare ourselves for things by learning new skills, then a lot of things become far less threatening.

We need to see change as exciting rather than threatening, the more that we adapt and change the more that we will progress.

Now do Exercise 53.

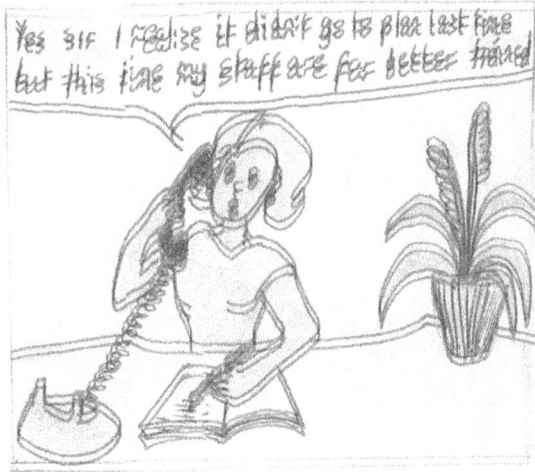

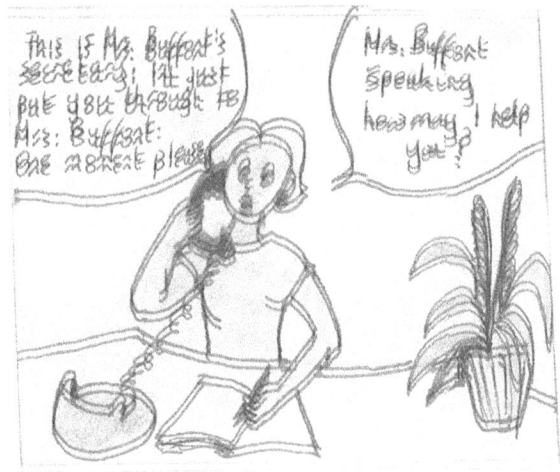

| Past experience helps you cope better with stressers. | You need adequate time to master and feel confident about performing new skills. |

EXISTING COPING SKILLS.

Past experiences and existing coping skills will help us to deal with some stressers effectively. If we have dealt successfully with a problem in the past it becomes far easier for us to deal with it when it comes up again, because we already have valuable experience and knowledge to help us. If we managed to successfully fit new brakes onto our car last year, the chances are that we will be less stressed by the thought of doing them again this year, because we already know what to expect and how to approach it. If however, we are asked to do something that we have never done before, something that we have no knowledge about, like say brain surgery, then the chances are that our stress levels will rise dramatically because we will not have had enough time to master the task before being expected to perform it adequately.

So prior knowledge, experience, perception, state of mind, skills already possessed and the amount of time allowed to master a new skill, all determine how much stress we will associate with any given task.

Now do Exercise 54.

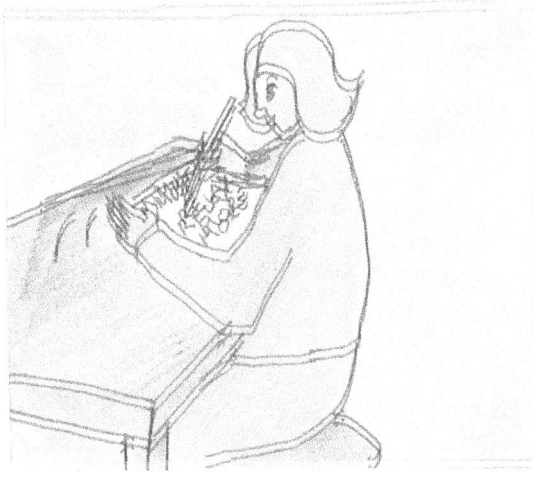		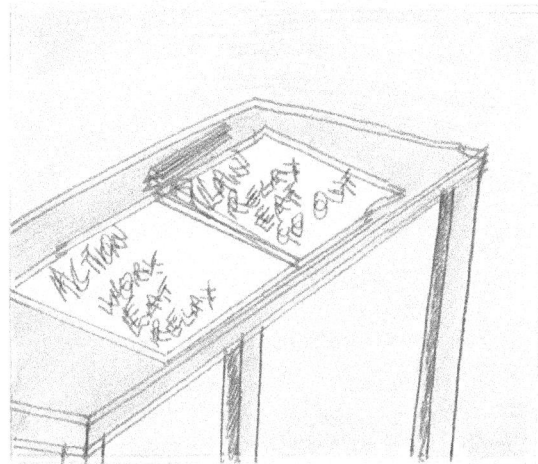
Write down any possible solutions to your stress on a piece of paper.		**Turn this list into an action plan.**

BRAINSTORMING YOUR PROBLEMS.

If you are being plagued by a problem that seems to have no immediate solution, try a process called brainstorming. Get a piece of paper and spend an hour writing down as many possible solutions as you can think of, no matter how ridiculous they sound at first. Remember wacky ideas can often be the seeds of sensible solutions. See if you can persuade any friends or family members to join in as well. Once the hour is over put the piece of paper away for a while. Then when you feel relaxed and ready, get out the paper and study the solutions that you all came up with. Cross out any that are completely impracticable and circle any that seem like reasonable ideas.

Eventually you should be left with a small list of possible actions that you can choose to take. The advantage of brainstorming is the fact that it allows you to uncover every possible option before making an educated rational decision.

Now do Exercise 55.

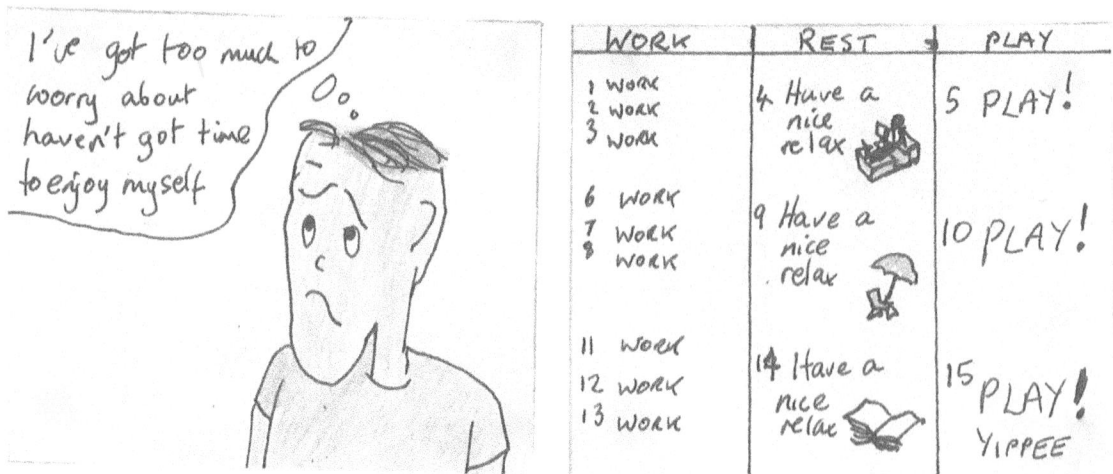

Do you allow yourself time for enjoyment?		Construct a timetable allowing equal importance to work, rest and play.

TIME MANAGEMENT.

When we become stressed about something, the cause of the stress (stressor) dominates our thoughts and actions at the expense of everything else. It is very important to keep everything in perspective. In order to remain physically and mentally healthy, you need to be able to participate in a wide range of activities that should all be considered as important as each other. For example, is working overtime really more important than taking your children swimming? Is DIY more important than actually enjoying yourself in the company of good friends?

The irony is that when we become stressed we seem to put less value on the things that help to de-stress us and more and more value on the things that cause us stress. If you can put together a timetable of daily activities, giving equal importance to work, rest and play, you will soon find yourself better equipped to deal with your ongoing stresses.

Now do Exercise 56.

84

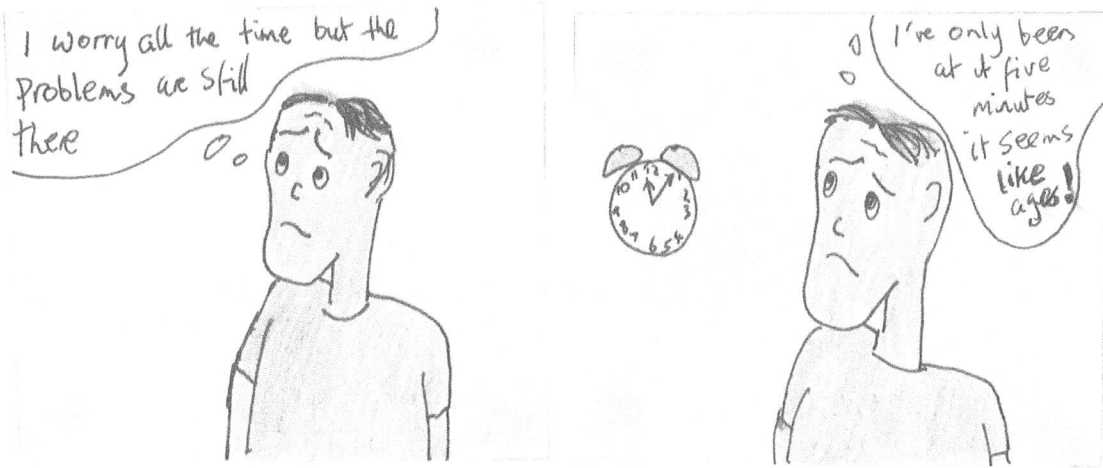

Does worrying all day ever solve your problems?		Try giving yourself a special hour each day just for worrying.

THINKING TIME.

When we are stressed we often find that the same old problems go around and around in our heads, dominating our thoughts and ruining our enjoyment of life. How often have you ever solved your problems when you are in this state of mind? The answer is probably never, so why waste all of your time worrying? Yes we may well have to find some solutions to our problems, so what we need to do is to try time tabling in one hours thinking time every day.

This can be our thinking time when we focus entirely upon our problems and look constructively for any possible solutions, or a time to formulate any possible action plans. Once the hour is over we need to stop thinking about it until our next thinking hour tomorrow. If at any time in the day we find ourselves drifting into worrying thoughts about our stressors we need to say to ourselves "stop! that can wait until my thinking hour".

Now do Exercise 57.

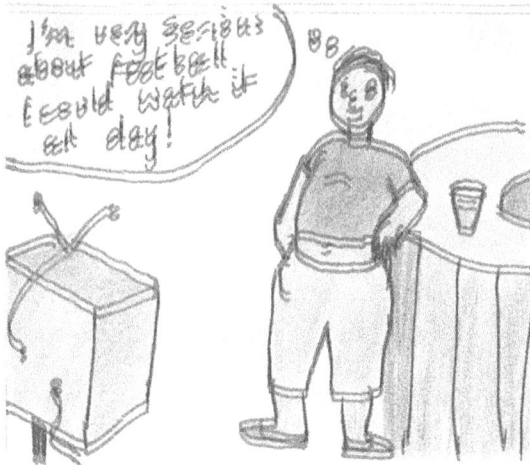

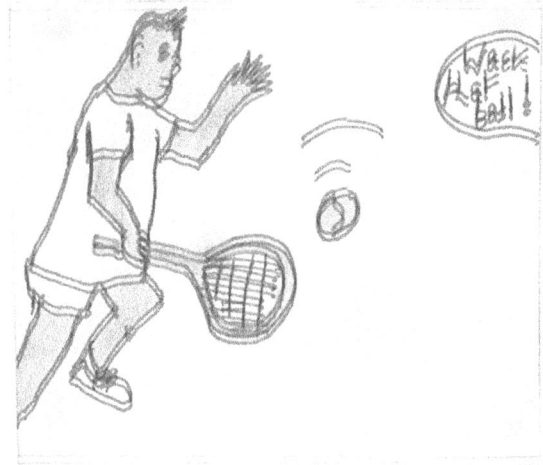

| How serious are you about regular exercise at present? | | Exercise can counteract a lot of the effects of stress. |

PHYSICAL EXERCISE.

Stress puts a lot of strain on our minds and bodies; regular physical exercise is one of the most effective ways to counteract this. Exercise increases physical strength, improves your posture, helps maintain a healthy heart, tones up your muscles, improves concentration, it helps you to relax and sleep, it helps maintain a healthy appetite, and it improves feelings of self-worth by generating vitality and confidence. It can also improve your opportunities for socialising.

There are many different sports that you can consider participating in and your choice will ultimately be decided by your age, state of fitness at present and the facilities locally available to you. The most important factor though, has to be choosing an exercise programme that you will enjoy; otherwise you will never stick to it.

Now do Exercise 58.

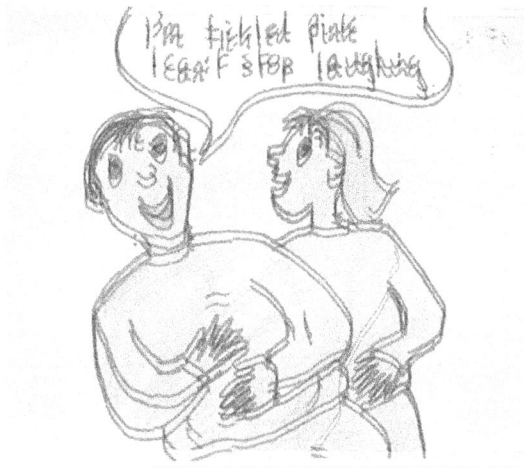

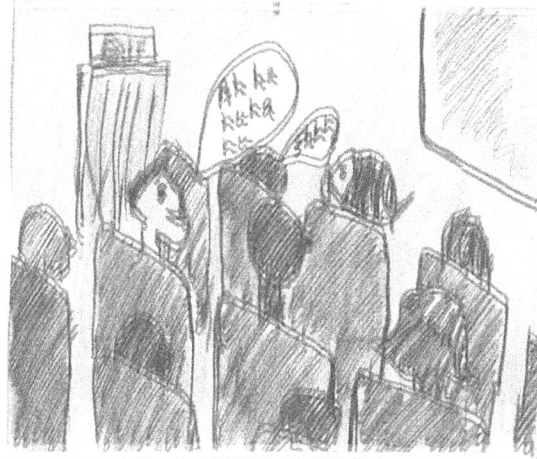

| Laughter can aid our recovery. | | Watch a funny film on a regular basis. |

HUMOUR AND LAUGHTER.

Seeing the funny side of things can often relieve stressful situations. There is now strong evidence to suggest that laughter can have a tremendous effect upon our well being. It has been known to stop deteriorating conditions in their tracks and reverses the process of the illness, thereby aiding the recovery process.

When we are depressed or stressed one of the first things that we lose is our sense of humour. If we are unable to find the funny side of anything, life becomes even more serious and stressful, making matters even worse.

Now do Exercise 59.

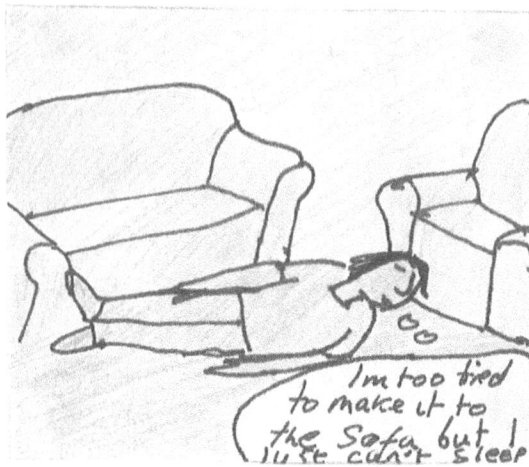

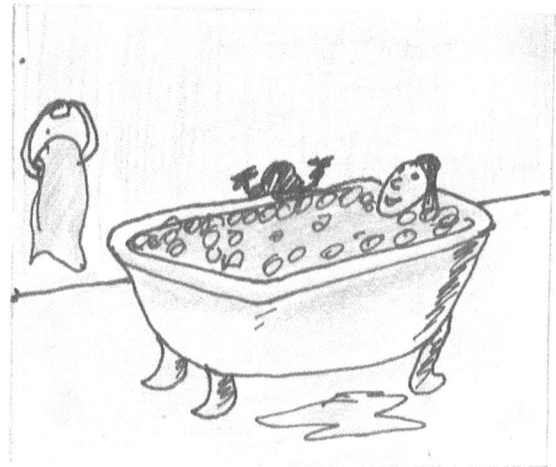

Lack of sleep can be very destructive.		Try to develop a regular routine when you prepare for bed.

SLEEP DEPRIVATION.

Sleep deprivation is very common among suffers of stress.   It can lead to deterioration in perception, reaction times, energy levels, memory, concentration and motivation. It can also lead to an increase in negative thinking.

If your sleep pattern is disturbed you need to think of ways to restore it. Look at patterns of activity before you go to bed, have they changed? Did you used to read in bed or have a hot milky drink? Try and get back to the way you used to be. Don't dwell on problems before bedtime, save them for your thinking hour. Try to go to bed at roughly the same time each night so that your body gets into a consistent routine. Try not to sleep too much in the daytime, as it will affect your routine. Ironically the worst thing that you can do is tell yourself that you must get to sleep when you go to bed as this will only make you concentrate upon why you can't get to sleep.

Now do Exercise 60.

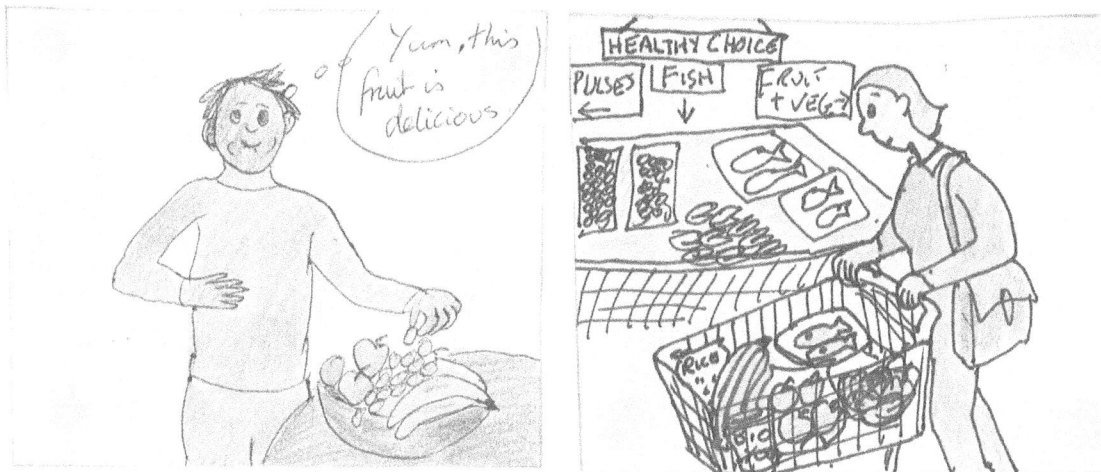

A healthy diet is vital when it comes to reducing stress.		Make sure that you stick to a healthy diet.

NUTRITION AND DIET.

A healthy diet is vital at all times but when we are suffering from stress it becomes even more crucial because our bodies need extra resources to help maintain the extra energy that they are now burning up.

When our nutrition is good our organs, muscles and tissues are healthy. Our energy level is high, our bodies are strong and resistant to the adverse effects of the environment, and our minds are hopefully clear. There are many books available on healthy diets so here are just a few general tips.

- Eat plenty of fresh fruit and vegetables on a daily basis.

- Eat fresh fish two to three times a week.

- Cut down on sugar and salt intake.

- Do not eat too much red meat.

- Try and avoid fried foods.

- Avoid snacking between meals on biscuits, crisps and chocolate bars.

- *Stick to using semi-skimmed milk rather than full fat.*

Now do Exercise 61.

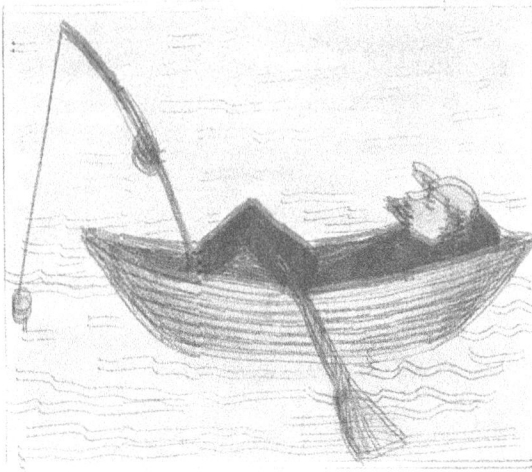

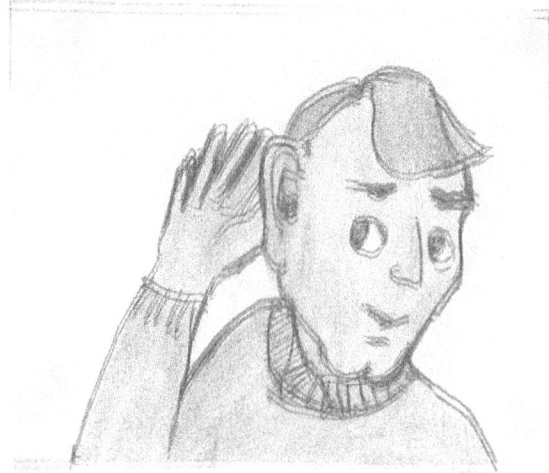

Encourage relaxing pastimes.		Become a sympathetic listener.

WHAT CAN FAMILY AND FRIENDS DO TO HELP?

It can be very difficult to deal with somebody who is stressed, they tend to be short-tempered, irritable, highly charged and anti-social. As a friend you need to be a calm rational influence upon them, do not allow yourself to get caught up in their level of distress. Use your influence to try and relax them get them interested in pursuing some relaxing pastimes with you, go for a country walk, play a round of golf, visit a teashop. Encourage them to enjoy themselves without feeling guilty. Do anything that will lower their level of distress and avoid anything that is likely to increase it, like busy traffic, crowded shops, etc. Try to encourage them to talk rationally about their worries when they are more relaxed. Become an understanding listener, offer advice but avoid criticism.

DEPRESSION

DRUGS AND ALCOHOL

ANXIETY

LOW

SELF-ESTEEM

ANGER

STRESS

POOR ASSERTIVENESS

To dislike other people
whom we cannot change
seems understandable and
a matter of personal taste.

To dislike ourselves,
who we can change,
seems an illogical notion
and a complete waste.

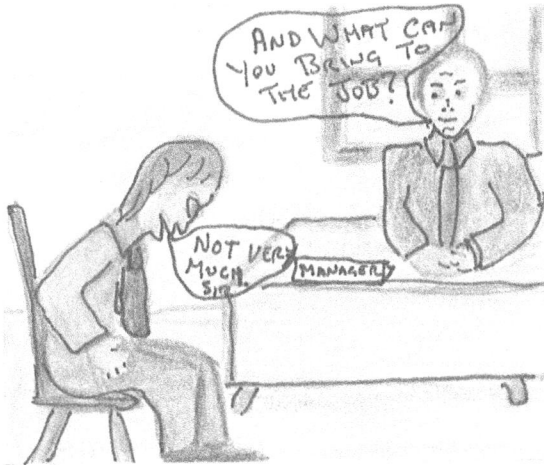

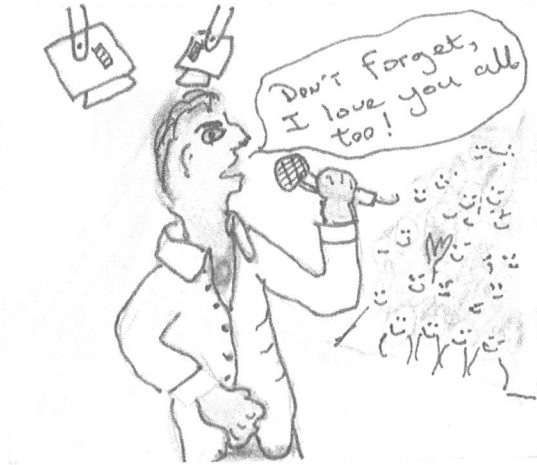

People with low self-esteem project the feeling that they do not like themselves.	High self-esteem puts us onto a positive spiral that can pull us out of depression.

THE LINK BETWEEN LOW SELF-ESTEEM AND DEPRESSION.

If we continue to have a poor self-image, we will soon establish a very dysfunctional belief system. We may start to see ourselves as unworthy people who are a complete waste of time and not worth bothering with. If we truly believe this we will project this image of ourselves across to others, who will then treat us accordingly. Their feedback to us will then make us feel even worse about ourselves and so we will, in essence, have created a spiral of negativity that can only lead us to depression.

If however, our self-esteem is high, we will value ourselves. We will see ourselves as a worthy person who is worth knowing, a person who likes themselves and a person who is comfortable with themselves. Again we will be projecting this image outwards to others, only this time they will be picking up on our newfound confidence and treating us with more interest and respect. The feedback that they give us will boost our self-esteem even more. We will now be in a positive spiral that can start to pull us out of our depression.

So self-esteem is clearly inter-linked with depression. The higher your self-esteem is, the better your chances are for recovering from depression.

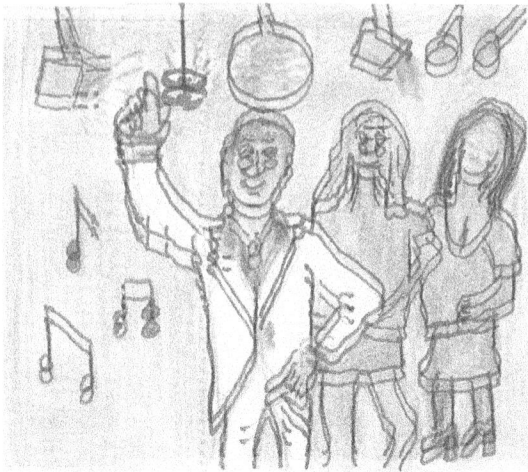

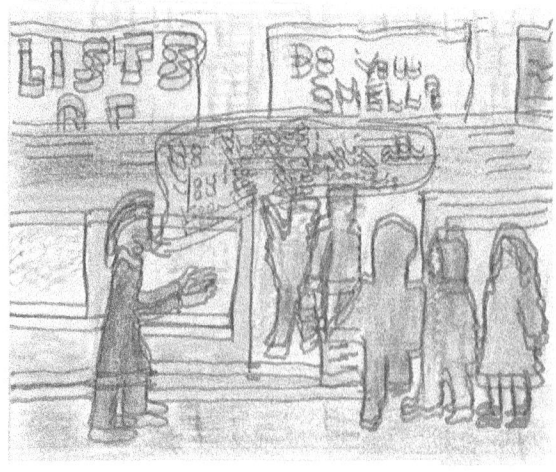

Self-esteem is the way that we feel about ourselves.		We might feel that others are far more important than ourselves.

WHAT IS SELF-ESTEEM?

Self-esteem is the opinion and respect that we have for ourselves. It is about feeling okay with the way that we treat ourselves, speak to ourselves and speak about ourselves to others. When people suffer from low self-esteem they are being very negative and critical about themselves, constantly putting themselves down and de-valuing any achievements that they have made.

Sometimes people behave in ways that deep down they disapprove of and this can cause them to feel ashamed of themselves. Sufferers of low self-esteem often believe that they do not deserve to be happy, that they are not as important as everyone else, that everything that goes wrong is their fault, and that they are being punished for being such a bad person.

Now do Exercise 62.

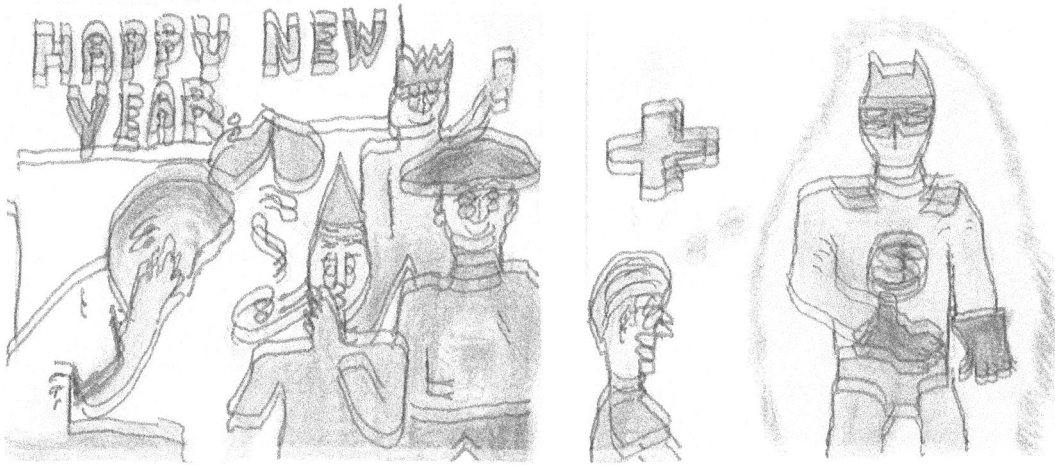

You are responsible for your own happiness:		Be positive and become the person you want to be:

HOW DO YOU IMPROVE LOW SELF-ESTEEM?

You are the only person who can take responsibility for your own happiness, so take time to start doing the things that make you happy. Start to respect your own time, health and enjoyment. Try to become the person you would like to be. Make friends with your feelings for our feelings and emotions can be a true indication of what we really want. You choose your own thoughts so if they are not helpful, change them for more positive ones. Remember, positive thoughts produce positive results and negative thoughts produce negative results.

Your biggest enemy is self-doubt and your greatest friend is self-belief. Let yourself be the best that you possibly can by releasing your full potential.

Now do Exercise 63:

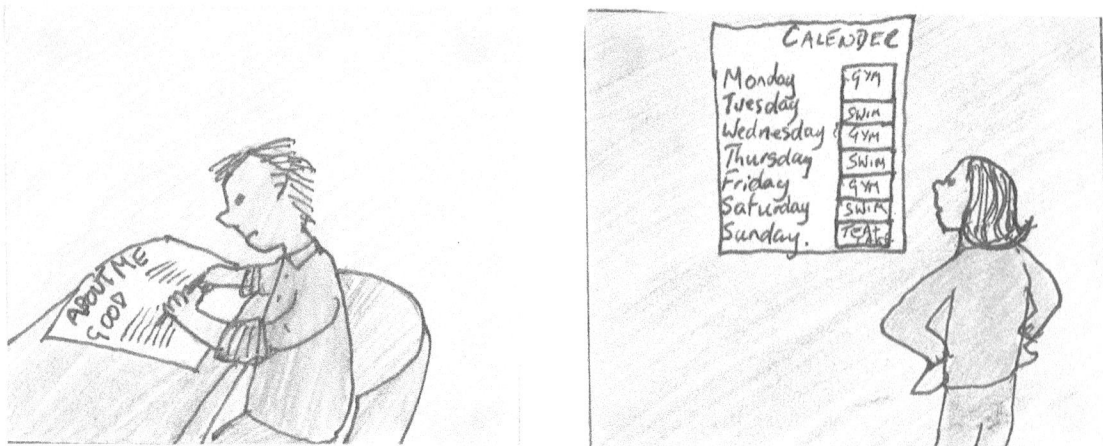

Make a list of positive things that you like about yourself.		Try to do something enjoyable everyday.

COUNTERACTING THE EFFECTS OF LOW SELF-ESTEEM.

We need to have some positive responses prepared and ready to use every time that we are plagued by negative thoughts about ourselves. Different people find different approaches more useful than others. It is important that you do the exercises below when you are feeling positive about yourself.

Now do Exercises 64 & 65.

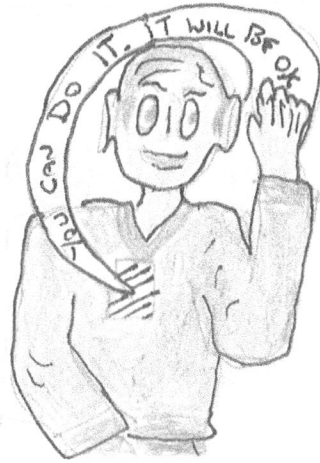

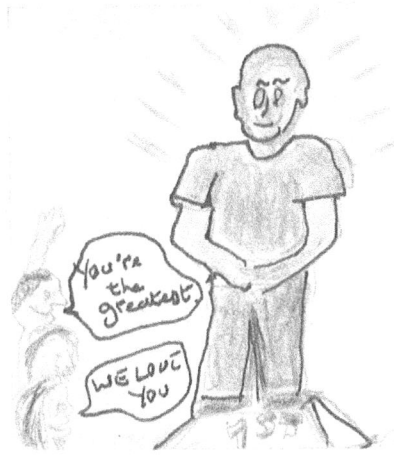

Start listening to your inner intuition.		Do not expect yourself or others to be perfect.

ATTITUDE AND INTUITION.

When we are functioning well our inner intuition guides us, it is almost like a guardian angel that warns us of danger and tries to guide us into making the right decisions. When we go along with our intuition we feel good, everything seems to slot together and feel right. When we go against our intuition things tend to feel wrong, we doubt our decision making process and worry a lot about possible outcomes. It is therefore important to be in touch with our inner intuition and respect the messages that it gives us. For our inner intuition is the part of us that knows what our emotions and feelings are really saying. If we can change our attitude towards ourselves, we will find that our other attitudes towards things will change accordingly. We can become more tolerant, accepting, loving and less critical of others and ourselves. If we can accept that we don't have to be perfect we can also accept that others don't have to be perfect either.

Now do Exercise 66.

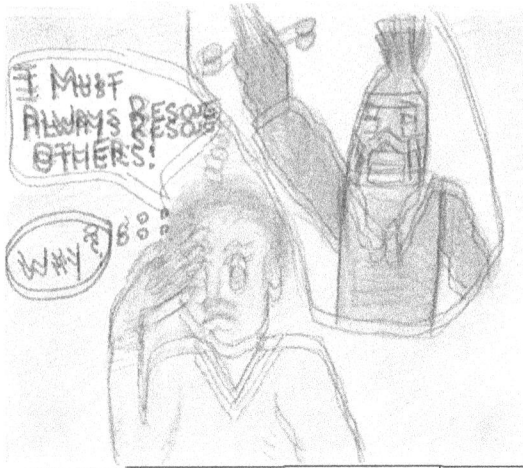

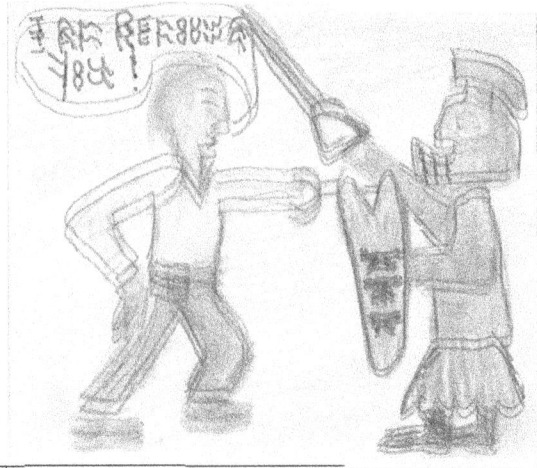

Identify beliefs that cause you inner conflict:		Learn to challenge these beliefs and if necessary remove them:

IDENTIFY IRRATIONAL BELIEFS:

If your self-esteem is low you are probably holding onto some entrenched irrational beliefs. Sayings such as "I must be successful, competent and achieving in everything I do if I am to consider myself worthy", or "the past is all-important, so if something once strongly affected one's life it cannot now be altered".

If you have and maintain such rigid views, there is a high chance that they will eventually cause you some difficulties and dissatisfaction. Learn to question the validity of any rigid views or beliefs that you have. Why do you think like that? Where did the view originally come from? What use does it serve now? Some views might still be useful and serve you well, so don't discard them just for the sake of it, make sure that you have studied and questioned them from all angles before making your decision.

Now do Exercise 67:

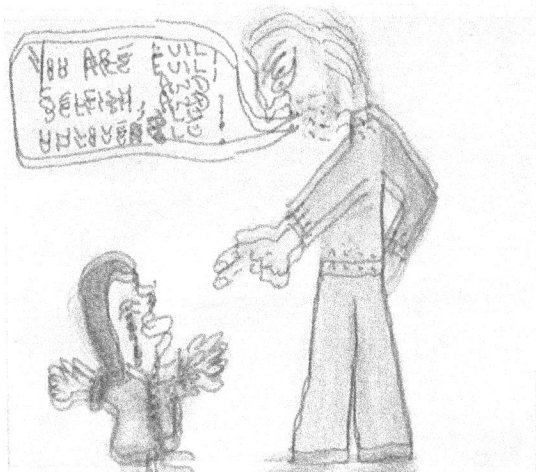

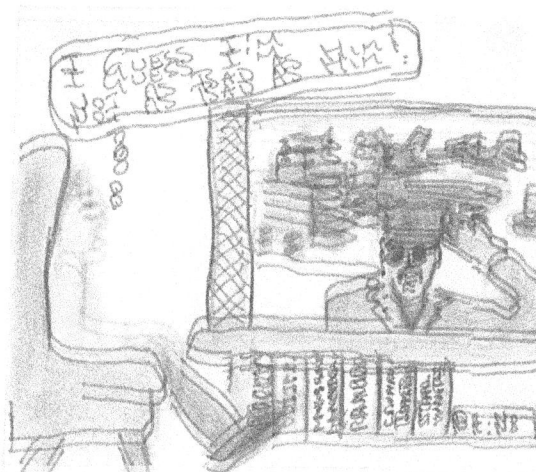

Negative messages were established in childhood:		Challenge the validity of these negative messages:

HOW IS LOW SELF-ESTEEM ESTABLISHED?

Self-esteem relies very much upon how others see us. The level is usually established in the formative years before the age of seven and it is dependent upon the messages that we receive from parents, teachers, siblings and peers.

As a child we believe that whatever our parents say must be right, so if we receive negative messages from them about ourselves, we absorb them and they become part of our personality. Of course no parents are perfect and so mistakes are often unintentionally made. As an adult you are now capable of challenging these negative messages because you realise that they are not carved in stone.

Now do Exercise 68:

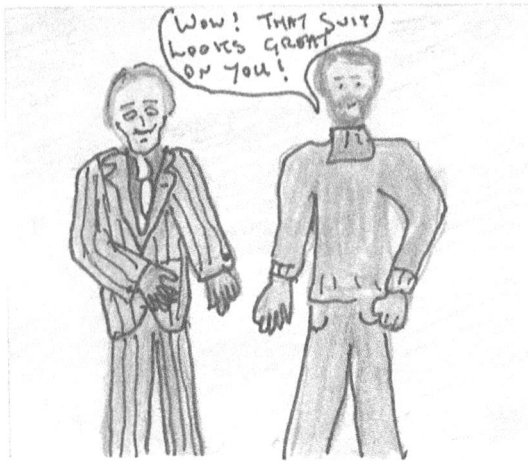

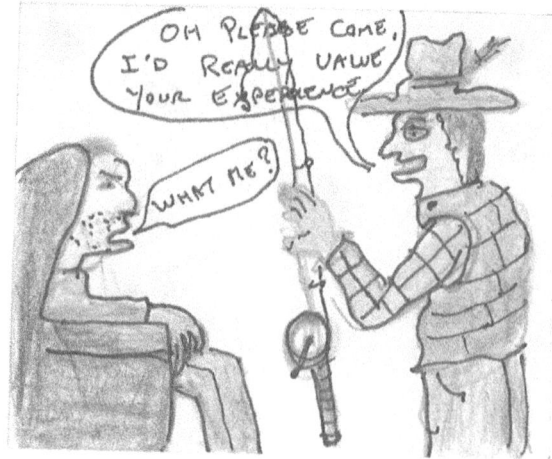

| Pay them regular honest compliments. | Encourage them to do positive things that they are good at. |

WHAT CAN FAMILY AND FRIENDS DO TO HELP?

Dealing with somebody with low self-esteem can be very difficult, as they will virtually invite you to put them down and support their view of themselves. You need to resist this temptation, try to give them genuine compliments as often as possible, even if they do try and reject them. The more you persist, the more likely it is that the compliments will eventually get through. Encourage them to listen to their own intuition and make decisions for themselves rather than relying upon your views.

Challenge their irrational beliefs; make them think long and hard about them and their validity. Get them to do things that you know they are good at, things that they will get some positive feedback from. Remain positive and optimistic whilst in their company, never undermine them in any way.

DEPRESSION

DRUGS AND ALCOHOL

ANXIETY

ASSERTIVENESS

ANGER

STRESS

LOW SELF-ESTEEM

To be given the gift of a palette of many beautiful colours,

Then to only ever choose to use one,

Is a missed opportunity and an awful waste of good paint.

Enrich your life by using

all of the colours

available to you.

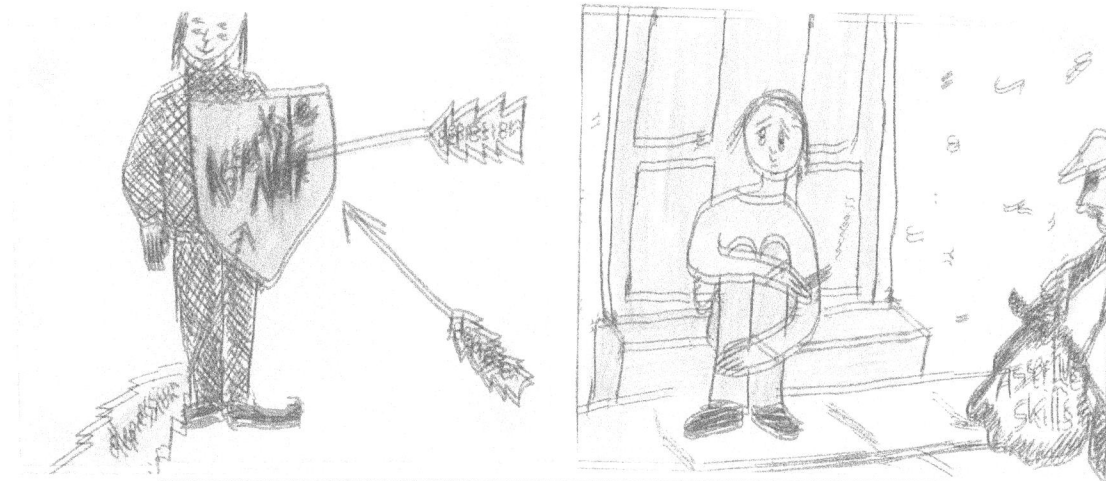

Assertiveness offers great protection against depression.	If you had all of your assertive skills taken away from you, you would soon become depressed.

THE LINK BETWEEN ASSERTIVENESS AND DEPRESSION:

If we are assertive we respect and value ourselves. We see ourselves as equal to everybody else and we are prepared to stand up for whatever we believe to be right. This approach is the best possible defence that we can have against depression, because it does not offer any opportunity for the symptoms of depression to get a hold of us. Yes, we will still get low in mood from time to time, but because we confront and deal with things as they happen we will not become entrenched in a backlog of unresolved issues. If we took away all the ingredients that make us assertive; being able to say no; being able to ask for what we want; respecting our own rights; having an insight into other people's emotions by being able to read their body language; having an understanding as to why criticism is necessary and feeling able and confident enough to express our own feelings honestly.

Take away all of this, and I think that every one of us would have just cause to become depressed. So assertiveness and depression are very clearly interlinked.

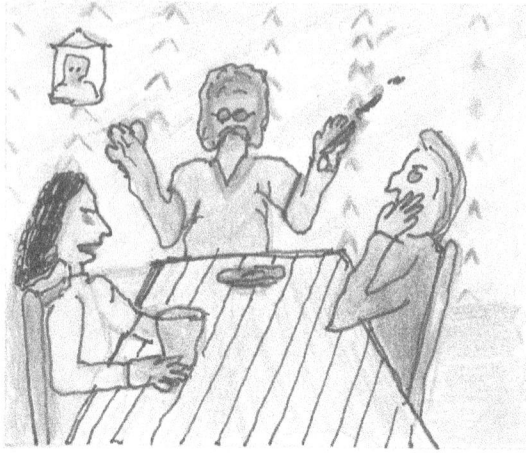

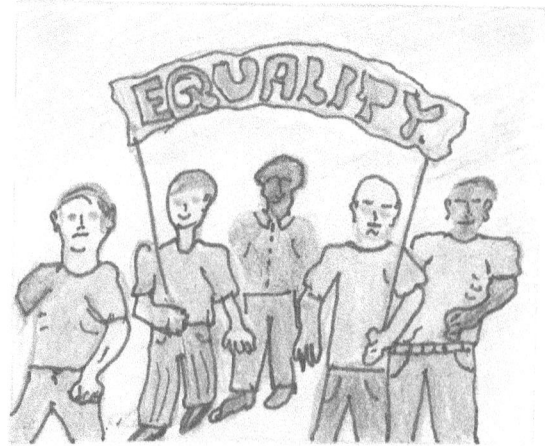

Is it about the way that we interact with others?		Standing up for our rights and believing in equality.

WHAT IS ASSERTIVENESS?

Whereas self-esteem focuses upon our relationship with our self, assertiveness focuses upon the way that we interact with others. If our interactions with others are dysfunctional, then we can lay ourselves open to developing depression, low self-esteem and anger management difficulties. It is therefore vital to learn about assertion for our own well being.

Assertive behaviour is about feeling able to express your views and opinions without fear of retribution. It is about feeling confident and safe to stand up for your rights when they are being abused. It is about being able to say yes when you mean yes and no when you mean no. It is about feeling able to make request of others without feeling personally rejected by their refusals. It is about being able to give and receive criticism without it leading to hurt.

Assertive people also recognise that others have exactly the same rights as themselves, so they always work towards equality and compromise in every situation.

Now do Exercise 69.

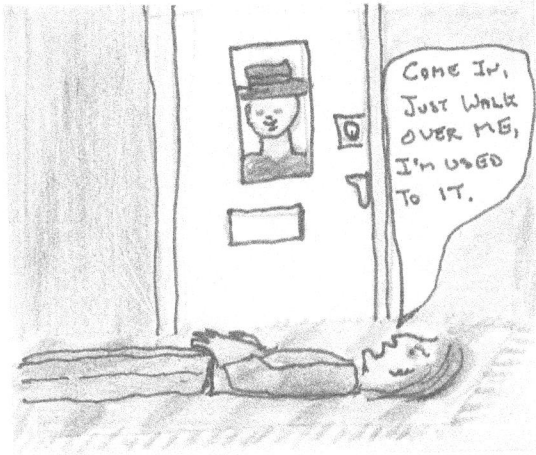

Passive people are known as doormats.		They se others as far more important than themselves.

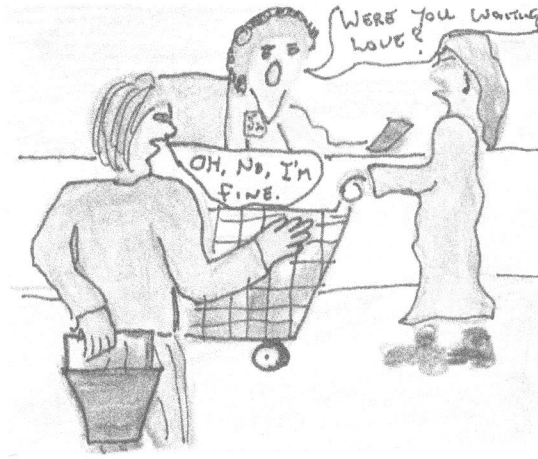

PERSONALITY TYPES.

In order to understand how an assertive person functions so well we need to first understand how other types of personalities function so badly. This should help us to identify how different personality types come across to others, what others will think of them and the long-term implications of such behaviours.

THE PASSIVE PERSONALITY – This is often referred to as the doormat syndrome, because passive people allow others to walk all over them. They feel afraid to stand up for their rights believing that everyone else must know better. They believe that the needs of others are far more important than their own needs. They do all that they can to blend in and avoid being noticed. In order to feel wanted they become over-helpful, often taking on too much for the sake of others. They struggle to make decisions, rarely offer a personal point of view and tend to say things in order to please others. The message that they give off is often referred to as "Your okay I'm not okay".

Now do Exercise 70.

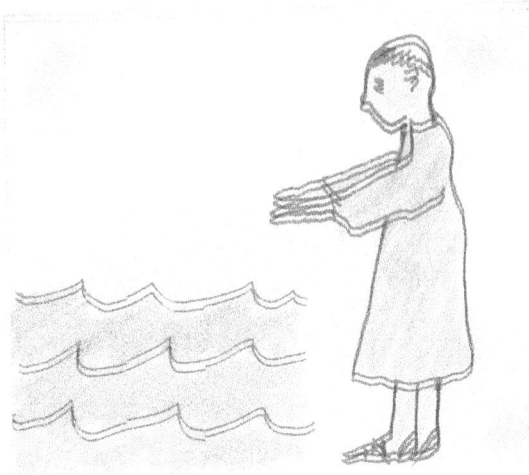

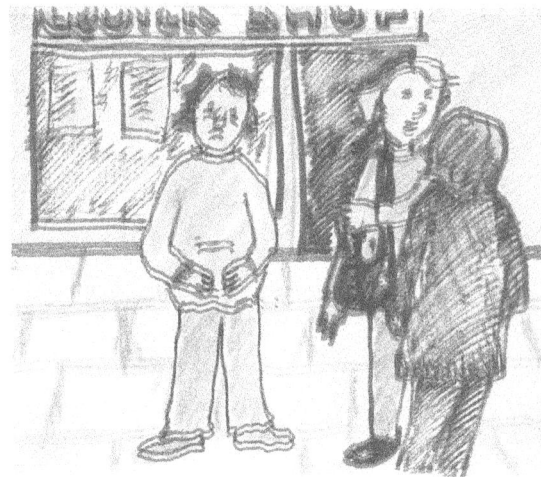

You are rarely blamed for anything because you try not to make waves.	Deep down you resent people's lack of respect for you.

THE PASSIVE PERSONALITY TYPE.

ADVANTAGES = you are rarely blamed for anything. You rarely offend people because you do nothing that could possibly offend them. You are considered a good sport because you are always helping other people out. You are thought of as an easygoing type of person because you never get worked up about anything.

DISADVANTAGES = deep down you resent the way that people take advantage of you. You feel that there is no outlet for your thoughts, feelings and opinions. Relationships are sparse and difficult because you are unable to express your true feelings. You feel weak, powerless and oppressed. Nobody really seems to value you or see your true potential. You run a very high risk of becoming depressed and because of all your built up frustration, you are the sort of person who can fly into an uncontrollable rage of anger when things really do get too much to cope with.

Now do Exercise 71.

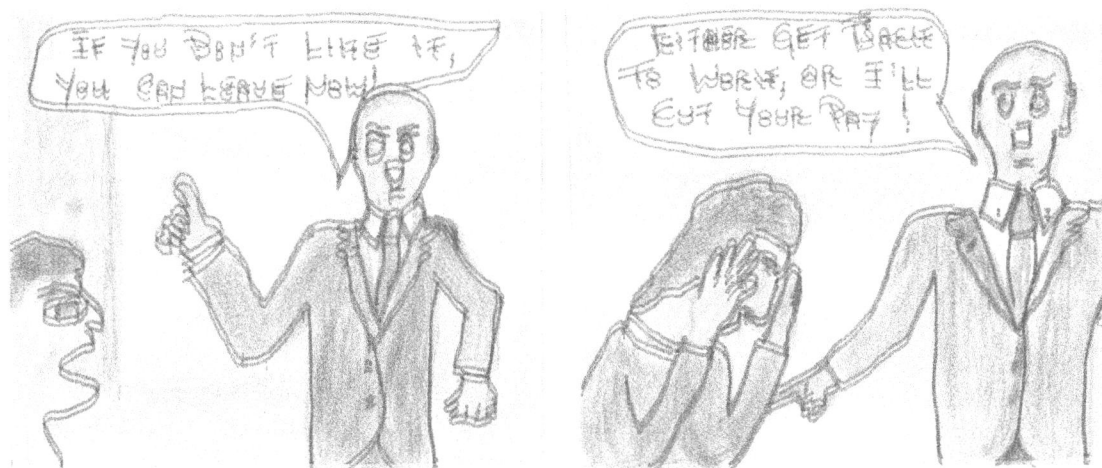

Aggressive people tend to rule through fear.		They have no interest in the feelings of others.

THE AGGRESSIVE PERSONALITY TYPE.

This is the sort of person who tends to be very bossy and domineering. They like to be in control and have no trouble expressing their thoughts and feelings about things. They have a strong desire to win and tend to view most situations in a win or lose context. This sort of person has no interest at all in the opinions or feelings of others. On the surface they appear to be strong and confident, but beneath this front lays somebody with very low self-esteem who can only boost themselves up by putting others down.

ADVANTAGES : You tend to get what you want, you have no trouble expressing your anger or disappointment and people tend to do what you tell them to do through fear. You may well be successful at work, as you are prepared to do whatever it takes to become a winner.

Now do Exercise 72.

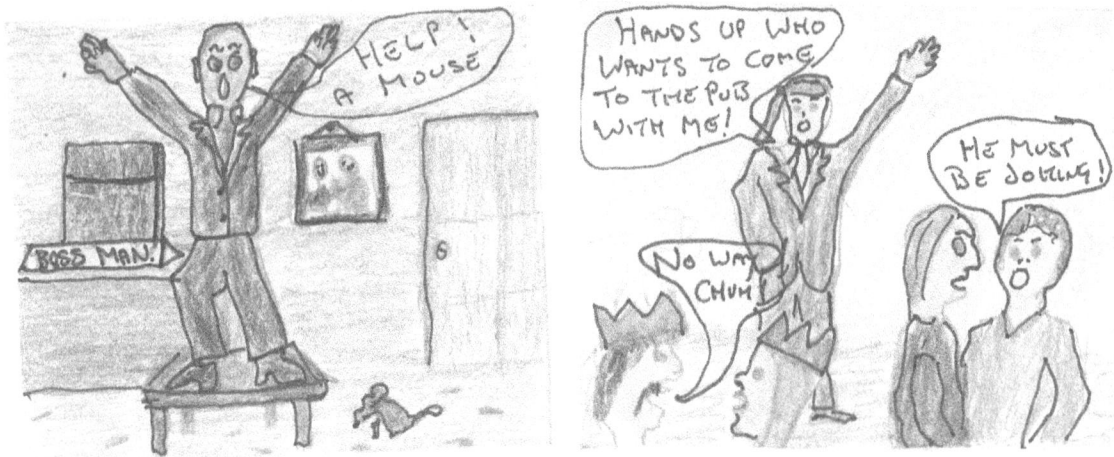

Aggressive people are really very afraid and vulnerable.		They tend to be disliked by most people.

THE DISADVANTAGES OF BEING AN AGGRESSIVE PERSONALITY TYPE.

DISADVANTAGES - Direct aggression is often a front for somebody who feels vulnerable and afraid of ever showing their true self. They may well find it easy to show their feelings of anger and annoyance, but when it comes to showing feelings of love and compassion they truly struggle. Sooner or later they come up against a bigger fish and when winning means everything, losing becomes devastating, destroying every belief that they ever held about themselves and leaving them in complete turmoil. It is also devastating for them to discover that very few people ever actually liked them, in fact most people would be more than pleased to witness their downfall with pleasure, after all the misery that they have caused them.

The message given off by directly aggressive people is "I'm okay, you're not okay".

Now do Exercise 73.

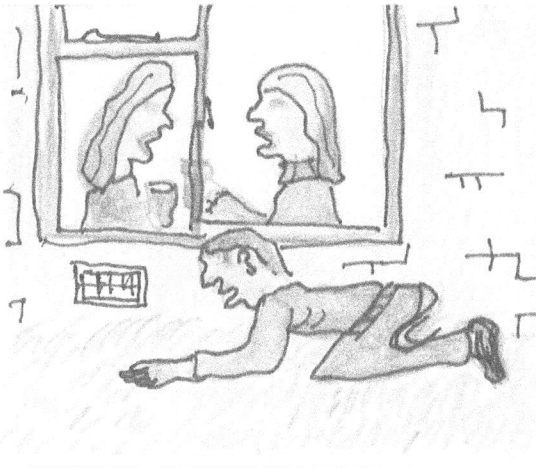

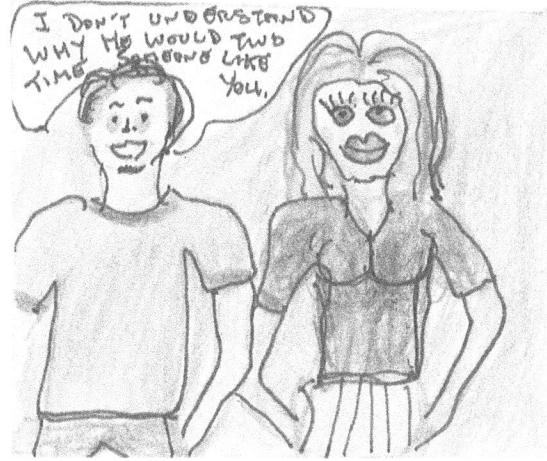

Indirectly aggressive people behave like sly foxes.		They try to control and manipulate situations.

THE INDIRECTLY AGGRESSIVE PERSONALITY TYPE.

This is the sort of person often described as a sly fox or sniper. They like to play mind games and manipulate situations to their own advantage. They always fire their shots from relatively safe positions, so that if confronted, denial is always possible. They like to make certain of an escape route before starting a fire. These are the sorts of people who will secretly slash your tyres for revenge rather than confront you face to face. They can secretly insult you by disguising their put downs with humour, or wrapping them up in what at first appears to be a compliment. They are difficult people to pin down as they always manage to turn the situation around, somehow making you look like the troublemaker rather than themselves.

The advantages of behaving like this include being able to secretly get revenge, never having to take direct blame for anything, getting others to do what we want them to, never letting others have any information on us that we don't want them to have and feeling able to manipulate situations to our own advantage.

Now do Exercise 74.

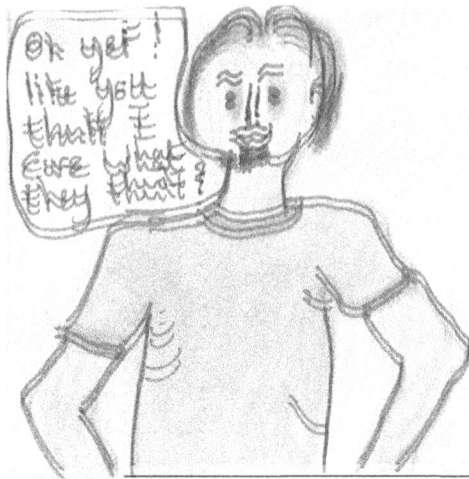

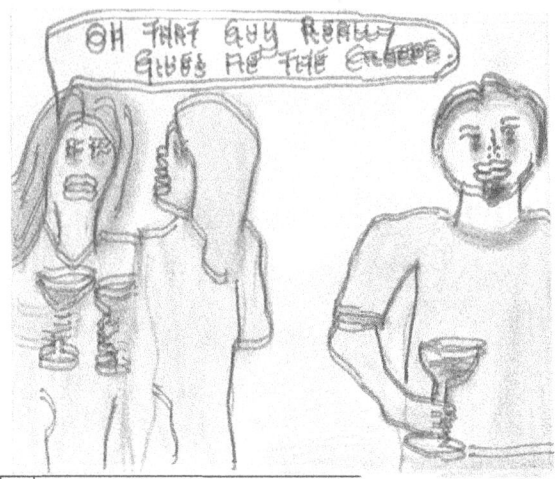

| Indirectly aggressive people never express their true feelings. | People can become very wary and uncomfortable around them. |

THE DISADVANTAGES OF BEING INDIREGLTY AGGRESSIVE.

The disadvantages of behaving in an indirectly aggressive manner include the following:

- Nobody ever trusts you.

- You feel unable to ever trust anybody else.

- You are scared to express your true thoughts and feelings because if anyone else like you got to know about them, they could use them against you.

- You can never develop close relationships because you are not prepared to reveal anything about your true self.

- Other people are very wary of you and may even reject you.

- Every situation comes down to a complicated mind game and power struggle that you have to win at all costs.

- This destroys your ability to ever switch off and fully relax.

Now do Exercise 75.

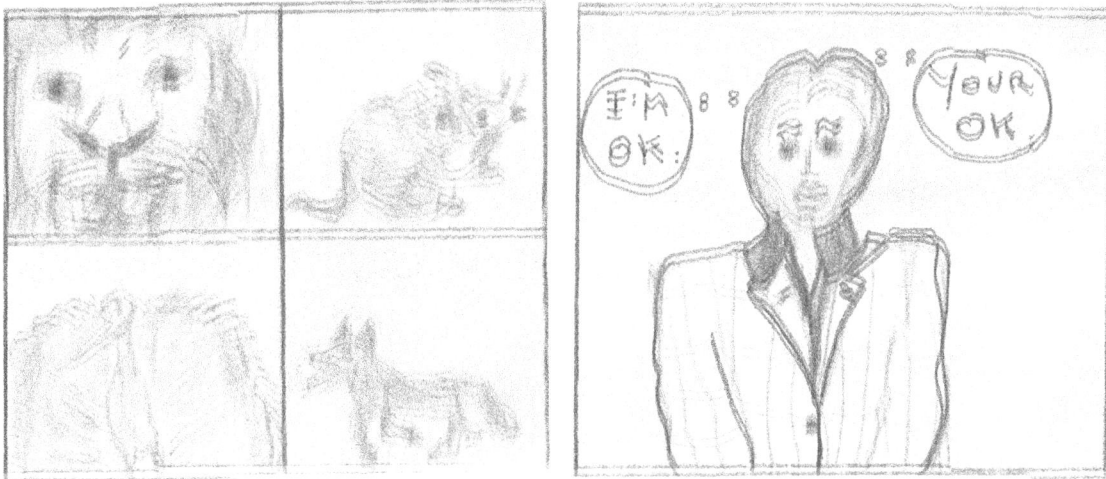

| We all use every personality type at various times. | Assertiveness is the most effective and least damaging. |

SO WHICH PERSONALITY TYPE ARE YOU?

By now you have probably managed to categorise a few people that you know into their behaviour types, but you are probably already thinking which one am I? The truth is that the majority of us fit into all of the categories at various different times. We can all behave assertively or aggressively when we want to, we might chose to be indirectly aggressive or passive in certain situations.

The skill that we need to develop is an awareness of how we behave and how that behaviour ultimately affects us. WE also need to become aware of the way that other people behave towards us and how that affects us as well.

From what we have just seen, behaving assertively appears to be the most beneficial way that we can behave in most situations. It is open, direct, polite, clear and honest. It gives us the opportunity to express our true feelings and show respect and concern for the other person's point of view, allowing both parties to work towards a compromise if an agreement cannot be met beforehand.

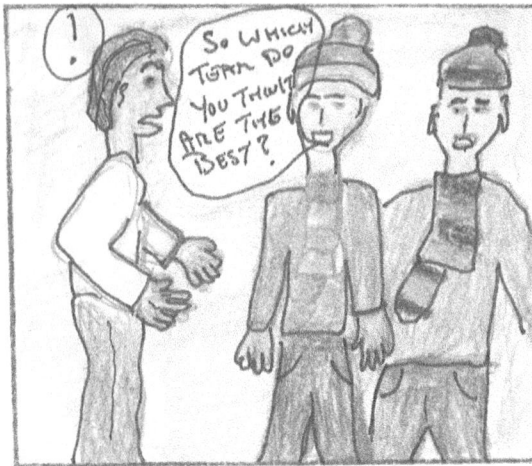

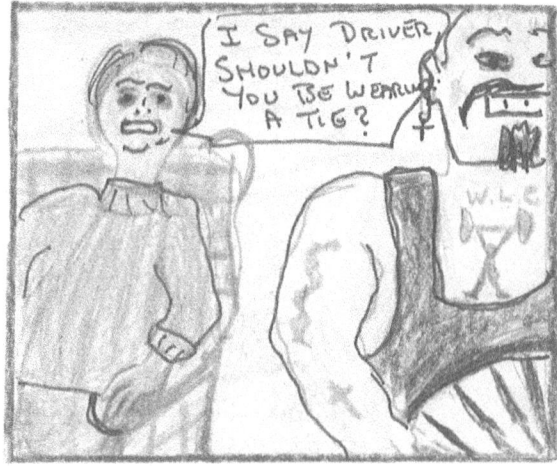

| We cannot be assertive 100% of the time. | We need to accept that in some situations being assertive could be very difficult. |

TRYING TO REMAIN ASSERTIVE IS NOT ALWAYS EASY.

The object of any assertiveness course is to increase the proportion of time that we spend being assertive, so that we receive more positive and less negative feedback about our own performance. It should equip us to deal better with people who try to make us think that we are dysfunctional in order to raise their own self-esteem. Nobody ever aims to make you 100% assertive because they know that that would not be either possible or desirable. Some situations may require a certain level of acceptance, we know that we could be assertive but we are prepared to accept the consequences of behaving passively or aggressively.

For example what happens if you have been assertive and worked towards a compromise, but the other person is still completely unreasonable? You would then have to either back down and decide to become passive, or you could choose to become aggressive.

Now do Exercise 76.

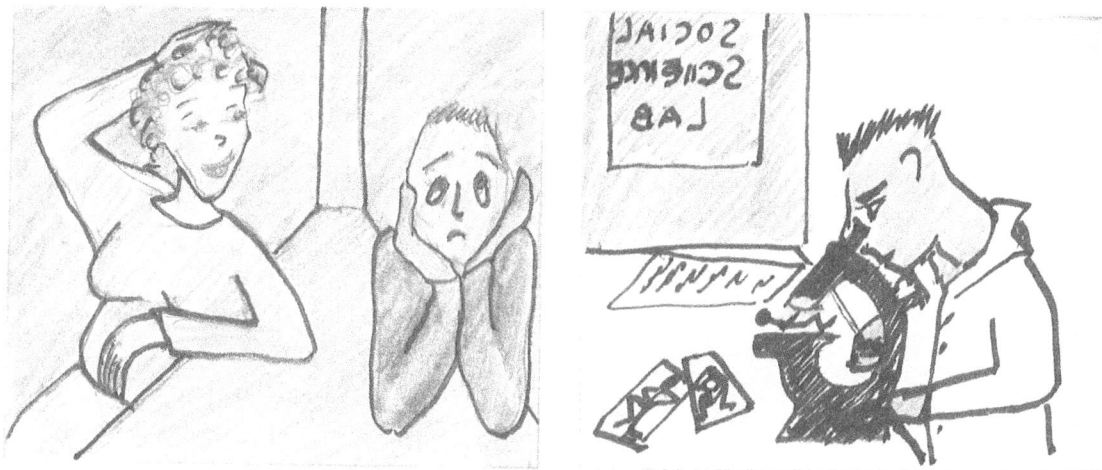

| **Body language can tell us a lot about someone's feelings.** | **Learning to recognise and understand it is a useful skill to have.** |

UNDERSTANDING BODY LANGUAGE.

We all use body language, some cultures are far more expressive than others are, but a lot of the basic assumptions that we use to gauge the mood and confidence of others are similar in every culture.

If we listen to two people conversing in a foreign language that is unfamiliar to us we tend to get more of an understanding about what is going on by watching their body language. We can also listen to the volume of their voices, view how closely they stand to each other and how open or how defensive they are towards each other. All of these things can tell us so much even though we have no understanding of the words actually spoken.

Being aware of your own and other people's body language is an important assertiveness skill.

Now do Exercise 77.

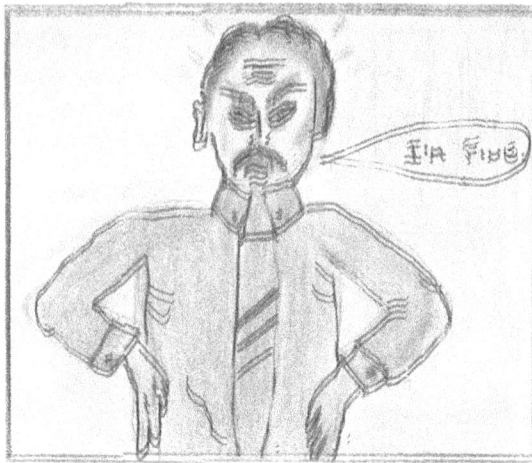

| Body language gives out more information than the words said. | How do you feel if somebody stands too close to you? |

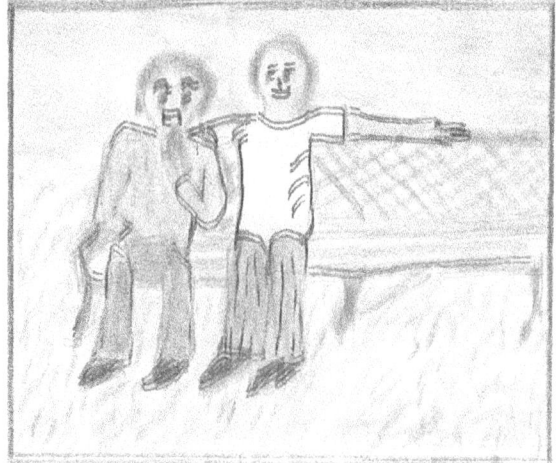

DECIPHERING BODY LANGUAGE.

The actual words used amazingly only account for 7% of the message we finally decipher. The way the words are said accounts for 38%. Body language accounts for 55% of the information we take in or give out! So it is clearly worth being aware of the effects our body language has on others and the effect that theirs has upon us. How do you feel for instance if somebody stands too close to you when they are talking to you? If anyone other than close family comes nearer than an arm's length, they are invading your personal body space; you will therefore immediately become defensive. You will feel threatened and vulnerable. You will not be listening to the words said because you will be preoccupied with removing them from your body space.

How would you feel if somebody asked you a personal question from the other side of a crowded room? You would probably feel exposed and vulnerable and would see them as completely insensitive.

Now do Exercise 78.

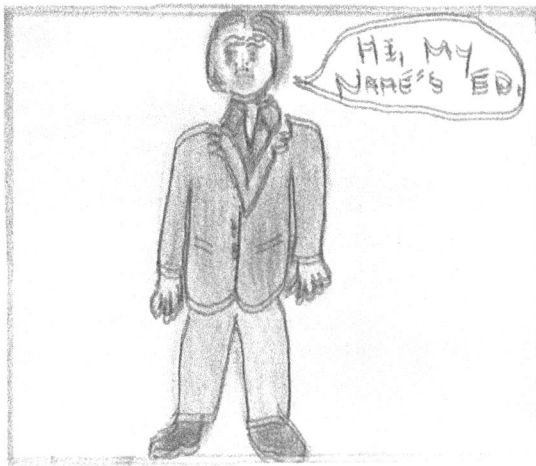

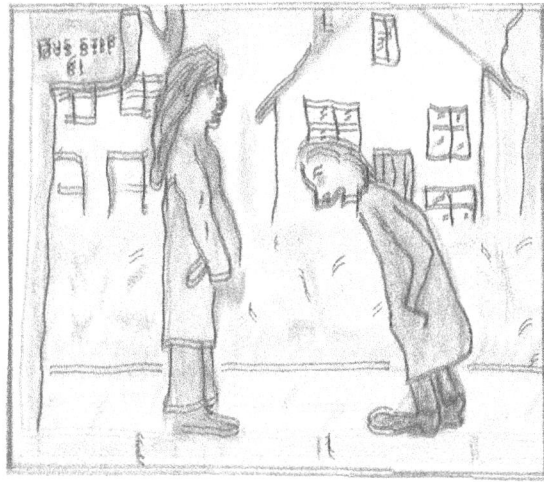

Stand tall and proud when you talk to people.		Look at the person and not the ground when you talk.

OUR IMPRESSIONS OF OTHER PEOPLE'S BEHAVIOUR.

What is your impression of somebody who tends to slouch down when they are talking to you? You probably feel that they are lacking in confidence. You should always stand tall, hold your head up high and try to feel strong and equal to others. How do you feel if somebody that you are talking to will not give you any direct eye contact? We tend to think that they are either trying to deceive us, or they are lacking in self-esteem.

What if they stare at you giving you too much eye contact? This can feel very uncomfortable, it either means that they are angry with you and are now staring you out in a threatening way to gauge your reaction, or it could mean that they are sexually attracted to you and cannot take their eyes off you. So always be aware of the amount of eye contact that you are giving. Try to use comfortable direct gazes, look people in the eyes when you talk to them, but avoid staring at them for an uncomfortable amount of time.

Now do Exercise 79.

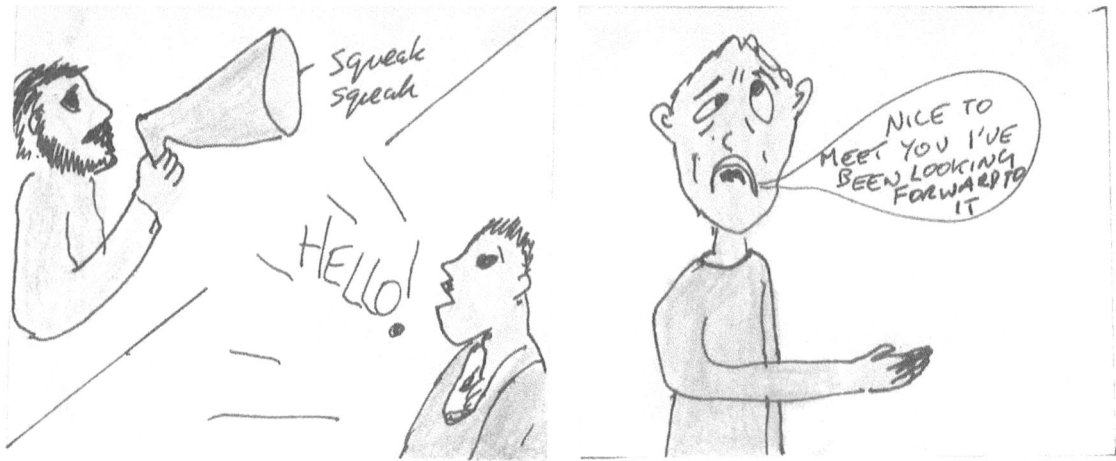

Be aware of your voice. Is it too loud or too quiet?		Make sure that your facial expressions match what you are saying.

USING OUR VOICE AFFECTIVELY.

We need to be aware of our voice; if it is too loud people will consider it to be threatening and aggressive. Their response will be to either avoid us or to confront us with aggression. If our voice is too quiet people will think that we are unsure of ourselves and that we are nervous, they will perceive us as being passive.

If our intonation is monotonous, people will find us boring, they will feel that we are not interested in what we are saying, so why should they be? If we try to keep a certain level of enthusiasm so that the intonation level in our voice can reflect this people will become more interested in what we have to say.

How do you feel if you are telling somebody something sad and they just continue grinning at you? Likewise if you tell them something funny and they continue looking sad? We tend to feel that they have not been listening to us. We need to remember that facial gestures are far more powerful than spoken words.

Now do Exercise 80.

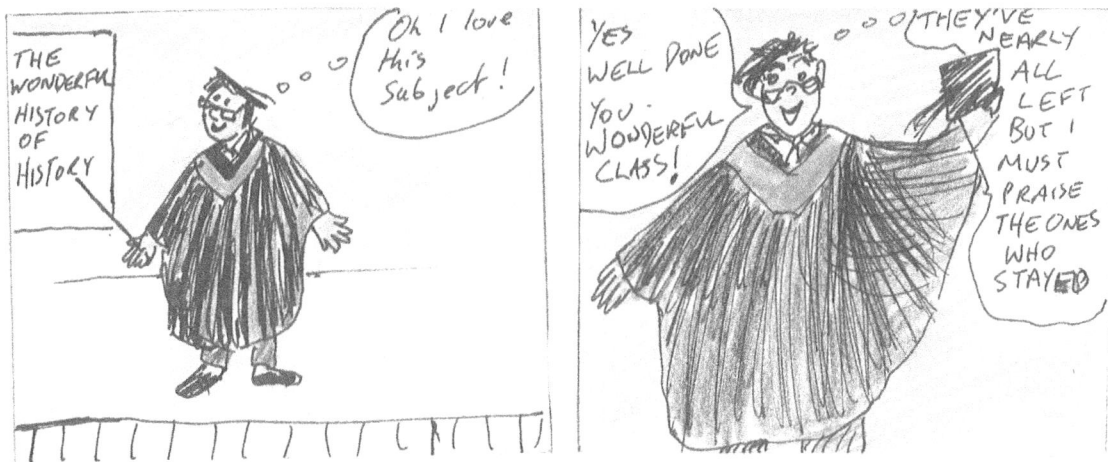

Owning and disclosing our true feelings can be very powerful.	It allows us to let things go without holding onto resentments.

DISCLOSING FEELINGS.

Expressing our true feelings can be a very powerful response. Most of us have learnt over the years how to hide our true feelings, but this can lead to problems. By using "I" statements we take responsibility for the feeling that we are expressing. These feelings can be positive or negative; the important think is that we express them honestly, without blaming other people for them. Instead of saying "You make me feel really angry when you behave like that". We can say "I feel angry when you behave like that". The difference is we are acknowledging that the feeling belongs to us.

If we are feeling particularly anxious it might be better to actually disclose this verbally, rather than waiting for people to witness us as gibbering wrecks. Once we have told them that we feel anxious, we can start to reduce our anxiety because we now know that there is nothing to be afraid of. Disclosing our feelings can be a very useful and powerful tool, even if it does not produce the desired result, getting our feelings out helps prevent a build up of negativity and resentment within us.

Now do Exercise 81.

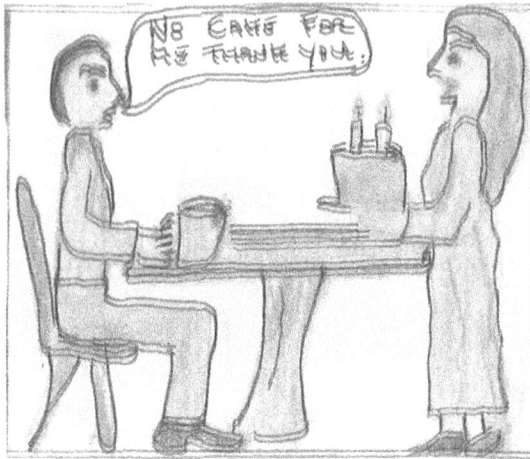

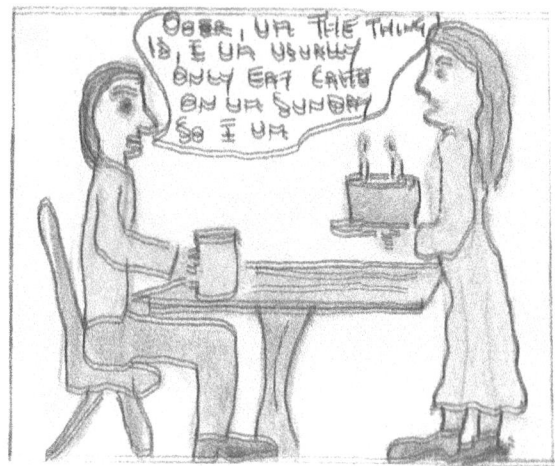

Always use short clear statements.		Avoid unnecessary padding.

BEING CLEAR.

How many times have you heard someone say "But I thought you were saying ......" after a disagreement? Misunderstandings are the biggest cause of dispute. The best way to avoid them is to be as clear, precise and specific as possible so that the listener is left in no doubt at all as to the meaning of your message.

Speaking in a way which communicates to others exactly what we mean is a fundamental assertive skill. When we are unsure about what we are talking about, we tend to pad out statements unnecessarily. This leads to confusion and misinterpretation. Stick to short, clear, precise sentences.

Now do Exercise 82.

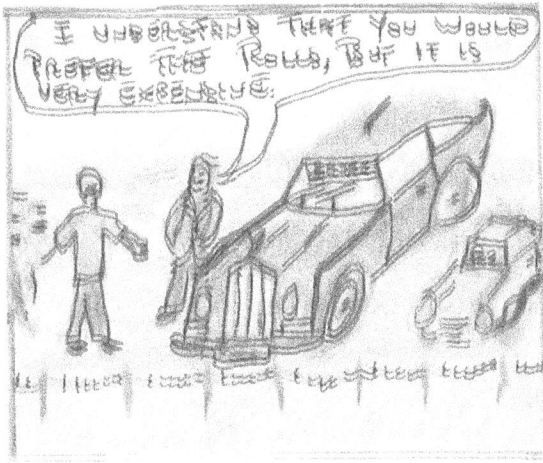

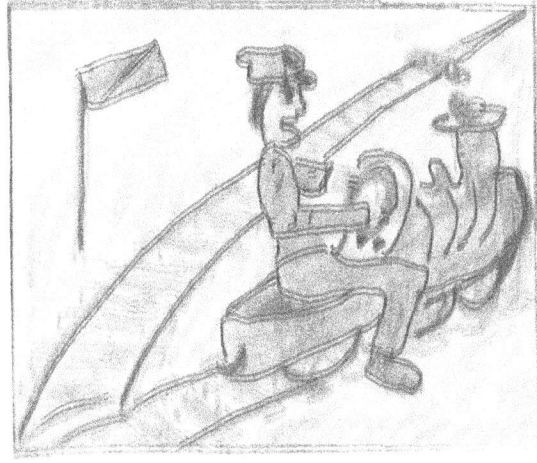

Show that you clearly understand their dilemma.		Do not allow yourself to be side tracked.

STAYING WITH IT AND EMPATHISING.

Staying with it is the art of keeping to the situation or subject in hand and not allowing yourself to get side tracked. Empathising involves showing a verbal acknowledgement that you genuinely understand and care about the other person's position. Used together these two skills allow us to avoid getting side tracked by irrelevant pitfalls and help us to work positively towards a resolution. For example, I have bought a brand new TV that keeps switching channels on it's own. When I return it the shopkeeper seems very stressed and keeps offering me a new washing machine instead, saying that TVs are the bane of his life. I say "I appreciate that the technical fault on this TV is not your fault and I am in no way blaming you for it, but I would like it replaced with the same model please."

See how I have demonstrated an understanding of the shopkeeper's dilemma yet also stated exactly what I wanted.

New do Exercise 83.

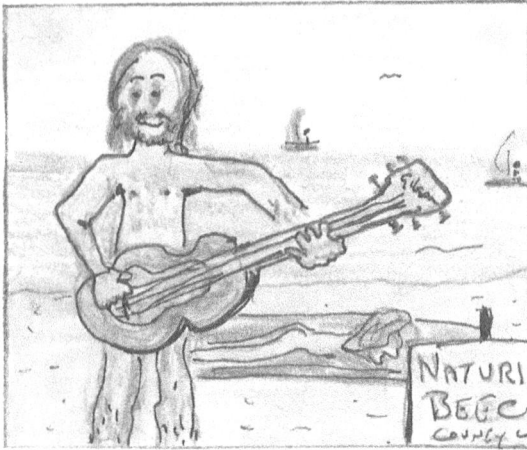

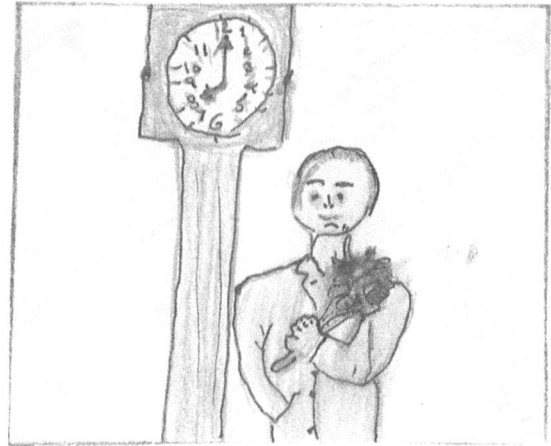

Prepare beforehand for awkward situations.	Use the situation to your advantage by choosing the time and the place.

YOU CALL THE SHOTS.

If you are faced with a situation that you know is coming up and you know that you are going to have to be assertive, use it to your advantage by being fully prepared. Clarify to yourself what you want to say and how you are going to say it. Wherever possible, you choose the place and the time to meet and make sure that you have a clear outcome in mind.

Sometimes we function better in the morning or afternoon, maybe the person we need to approach has good times when they are less busy and bad times when they are particularly stressed. IF you are returning something to a shop, pick a quiet time; always give yourself the maximum opportunity for success so that you will not look back upon the situation with any regrets. Then even if you fail to get what you want, at least you will know that you have given it your best shot.

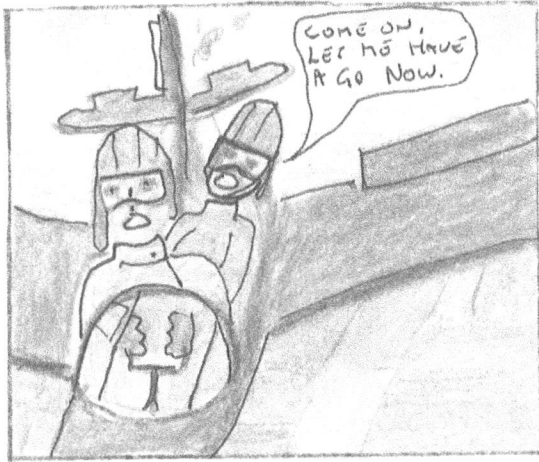

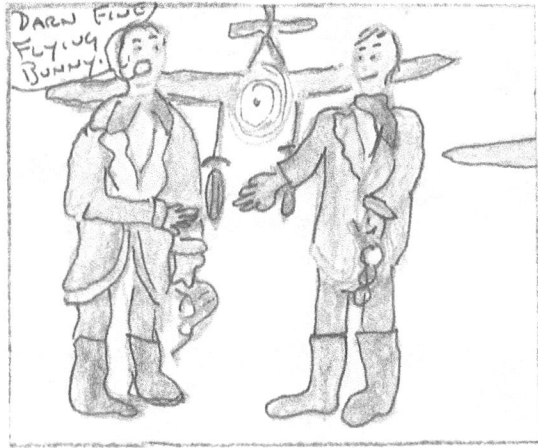

As developed civilised people, we need to be able to compromise	Compromise should leave both parities feeling satisfied with the outcome.

COMPROMISE.

One of our greatest assets as a developed species, that sets us apart from the rest of the animal kingdom, is our ability to compromise. So much of life seeks to be about winning, but if we can actually come away from a conflicting situation leaving both parties satisfied, that surely has to be a positive thing. Appreciating and empathising with the other person's point of view, whilst respecting yourself and your own point of view, is an essential assertive skill that we can all learn to appreciate.

Working towards an effective compromise is an effective means of reaching a solution and avoiding a stalemate or further conflict.

It is a mature reasonable approach that needs to be adopted and used far more throughout the world. People who are not prepared to compromise are considered stubborn, unreasonable and dangerous.

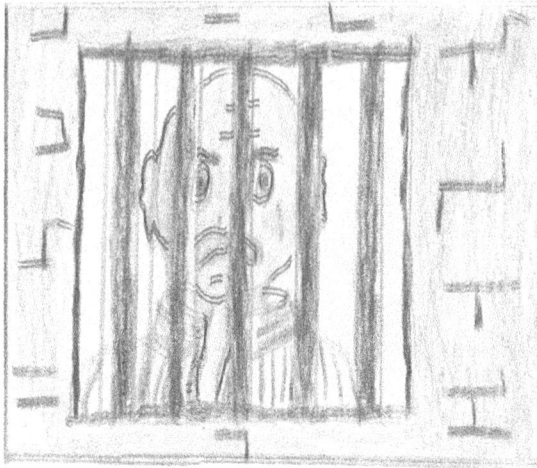

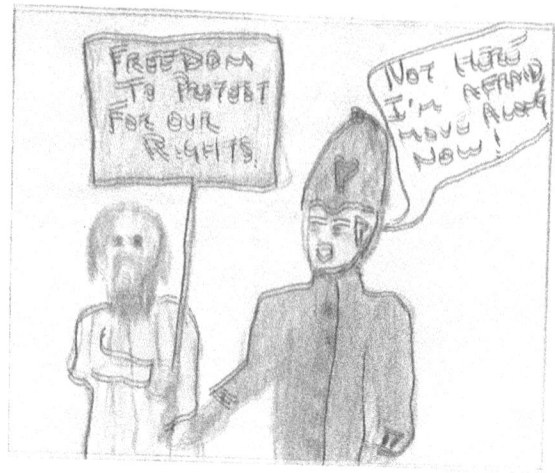

| We should all have a set of basic human rights. | | Without rights, assertiveness would not be able to exist. |

OUR RIGHTS.

The whole philosophy of assertiveness is based upon the assumption that we all have certain basic human rights. Aggressive people violate the rights of others. Passive people allow their rights to be violated. While assertive people stand up for their own rights whilst respecting the rights of others.

So how do we know when our rights are being violated? Because if we don't know what our rights are, how will we ever recognise when our rights are being denied?

Clearly not all countries allow their citizens the same rights and not all employers offer their workers the same rights and not all families allow their members the same rights. So we have to accept that the world is not an equal place. Even so, if we don't establish a set of basic ground rules that we would hope to apply to everyone, we cannot hope to ever really improve things for the better.

Now do Exercise 84.

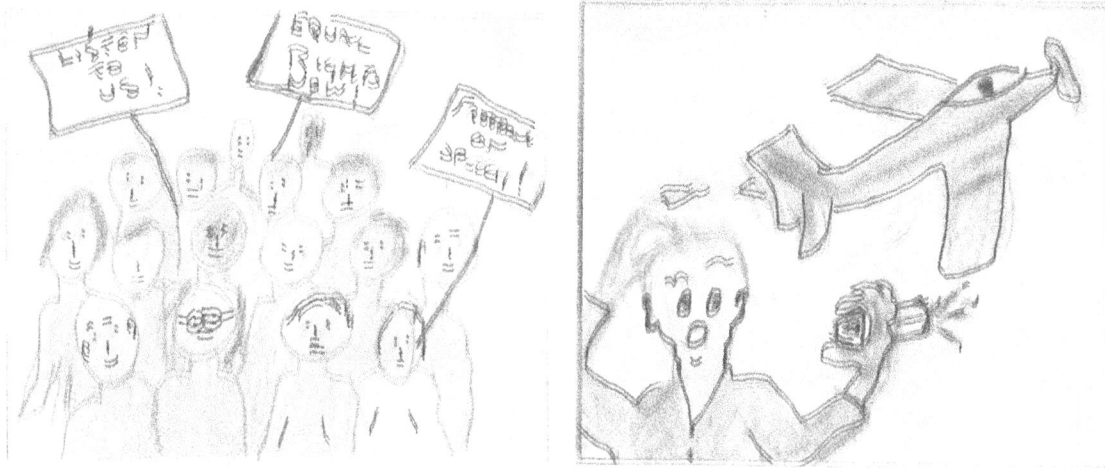

I have the right to equality and free speech.		I have the right to make mistakes.

SOME RIGHTS TO CONSIDER.

Here are some rights that should apply to everyone. Do you agree with them all?

- I have the right to be treated with respect as an equal human being.

  Does this always apply? Do you give more respect to some people than you do to others?

- I have the right to express my thoughts, feelings and opinions.

  Do you do this in every situation? How do you feel if you are not allowed to? Do you ever deny this right to anyone else?

- I have the right to make mistakes.

  Do you allow yourself this right? Do you allow other people to make mistakes? Do you think that we learn through our mistakes?

- I have the right to acknowledge my needs as being equal to the needs of others.

  Do you sometimes put yourself first? Or perhaps you tend to put others first. If we do not see ourselves as equal then we must consider ourselves either

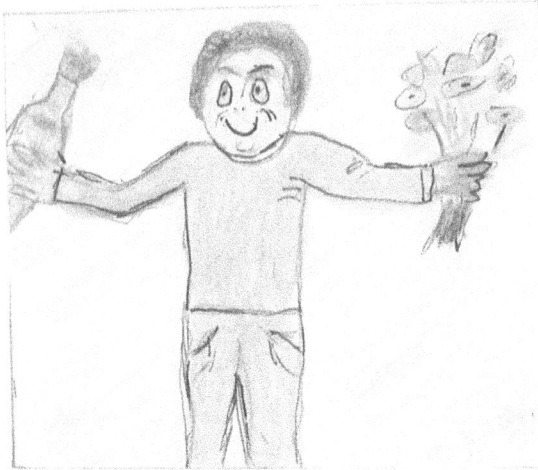

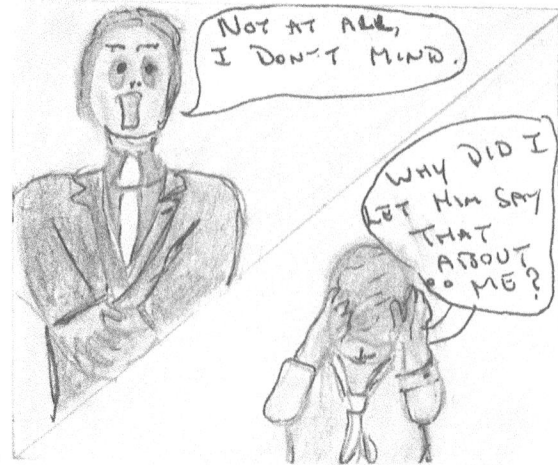

Learn to express your feelings.		It should help you to make the most out of your life.

OUR FEELINGS.

We are often brought up learning to deny our true feelings. Some feelings are categorised as bad feelings, such as anger and jealousy. We have been told that it is wrong and weak to ever show them. Unfortunately this is completely untrue; repressing feelings can be far more destructive. For example if we repress our feelings of anger it can lead to chronic depression. Being in touch with our feelings is a positive thing, they are there to guide us so we shouldn't see them as good or bad feelings, they are all just feelings that we need to act upon.

If you are unsure of your feelings try to get in touch with your physical, sensations they are all interconnected. For instance, if you feel a flow of warmth together with surging and relaxed muscles, the chances are you are feeling happy. If you feel tearful and heavy, you are probably feeling depressed. Remembering our right to share feelings and not being scared to take responsibility for them is an essential aspect of assertive communication.

Now do Exercise 85.

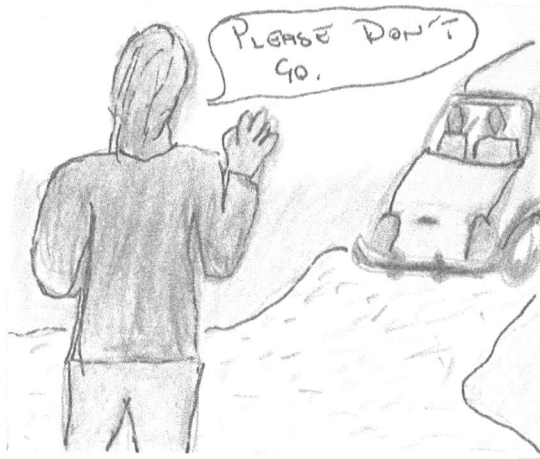

If we say no, we might risk losing friends.		Challenge your old beliefs and fears.

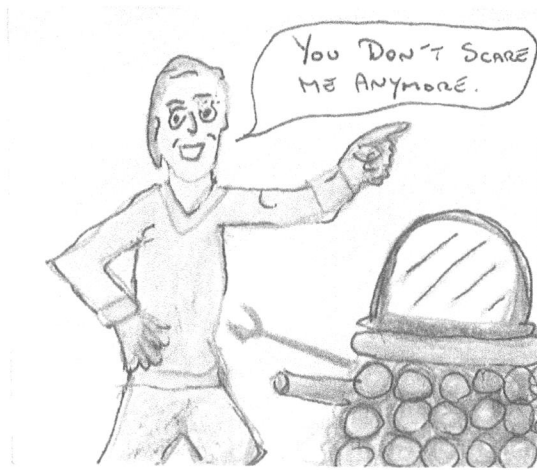

LEARNING TO SAY NO.

A lot of people struggle to say no, due to the strength of the underlying belief beneath the feeling. We might feel that saying no is rude or impolite, we might think that people will view us as selfish or unlovable. We might be afraid that we will hurt their feelings or we might ultimately fear being rejected.

We need to challenge these beliefs so that we don't fall into the trap of never being able to say no. How about replacing your old beliefs with the following:

- "By looking after myself I am better prepared to be able to look after others that really need me".

- I can choose to help others only if I wish to".

- "I am not responsible for other people's feelings".

Although it may take some time and practice to change your current thinking; your self-respect will soon start to rise as will the respect that you receive from true friends.

Now do Exercise 86.

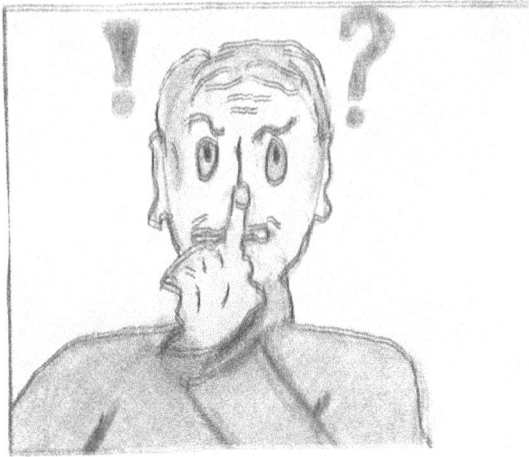

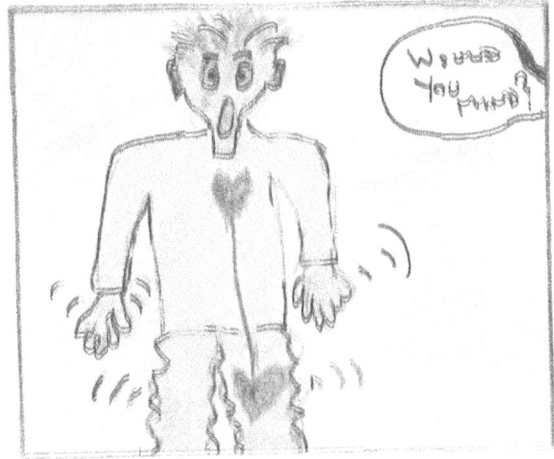

Why are we saying no?		Your physical feelings will give you an honest guide to the request.

PREPARING TO SAY NO.

Before we say "no" to anyone we need to have a clear idea of our own personal limits. Are they asking us to do something that we might actually enjoy? Are we otherwise engaged at that time anyway? Do we agree with what they have asked us to do? How long do they expect us to help them for? Will we get paid for it? Is anybody else able to do it? These are the sort of questions that we need to be asking.

We also need to be in touch with our physical feelings; do our hearts sink when the request is made? If so, then it is something that we are clearly unhappy about doing. Do we feel excited by the request? If so then it must be something that we want to do. If there is no noticeable reaction then the chances are that we do not mind either way. When we say "no" we need to make sure that we clearly use the word "no" in our sentence. We can offer a clear explanation as to why we are rejecting the request. (Not the person), and we need to make sure that our body language compliments what we are saying.

New do Exercise 87.

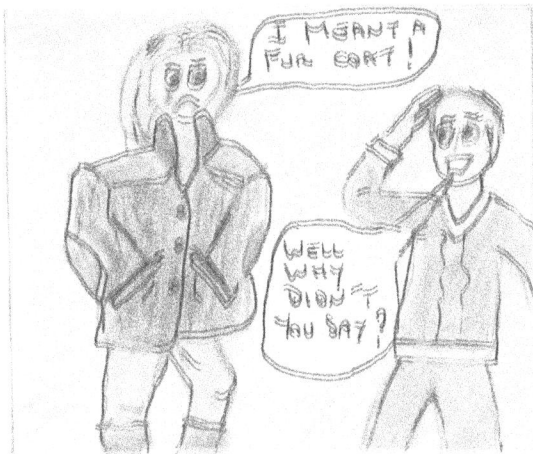

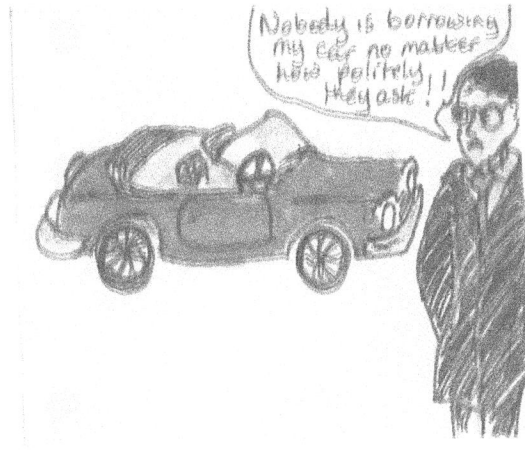

Just dropping hints can produce poor results.		Accept that is the request being rejected and not you.

MAKING REQUESTS.

If we never ask for what we want how can we expect others to know what we would like. Yet this is how a lot of us tend to behave. We drop hints and clues, we say things like "They should have known what I'd like", or "I tried to make it as obvious as possible". Why has asking for what we want been reduced to this ridiculous guessing game? Surely life would be a lot easier if we all felt able to ask for what we want, clearly and directly. After all you wouldn't go up to an ice cream seller and expect him to guess what flavour you would like would you?

The reason we find it so hard to ask for anything directly is because we fear being rejected. If we just drop subtle hints then the indirectly aggressive part of us can always deny that the request was ever our true intention. If, however, we ask for something clearly and directly, we have no escape route.

The answer is to accept that not all requests will be met, but when they are rejected it is the request, not you, that is being rejected. If we never make requests, then we will never get what we want.

Now do Exercise 88.

127

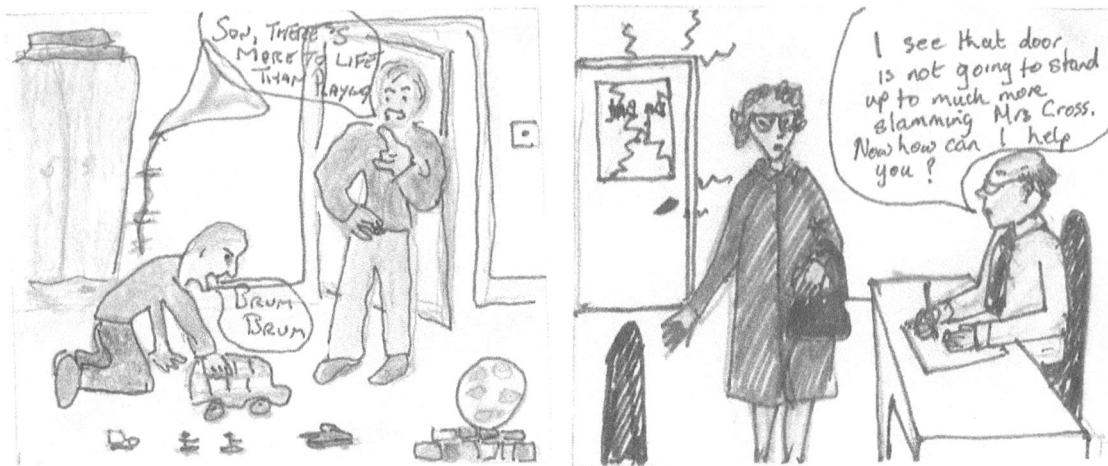

Criticisms that we remember receiving as children can still be upsetting today.	We should be criticised for the act, not as a whole person.

RECEIVING CRITICISM.

Why is being criticised always so painful? It is useful to recall childhood memories of the criticisms aimed at us then in order to understand what is going on now. As children most criticisms aimed at us would have been given to us in the form of a malicious put-down. "You're fat", "You're an idiot", "You're hopeless", "You're a wimp". Notice how these criticisms are aimed at the whole person, we are not told "That was a stupid thing to do", which only critics the act. Instead we are being told that we are a completely stupid person.

When we are given messages like these during our childhood we can take them onboard as fact. As adults we still remain vulnerable to such criticisms because we have never challenged their validity and so deep down we still believe them to be true. Criticisms that seem to really hurt are often referred to as our crumple buttons. Somebody unwittingly calls us an idiot, and it brings back a gush of raw feelings from the past.

Now do Exercise 89.

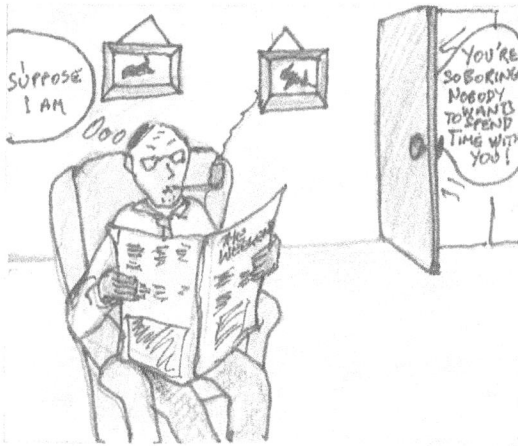

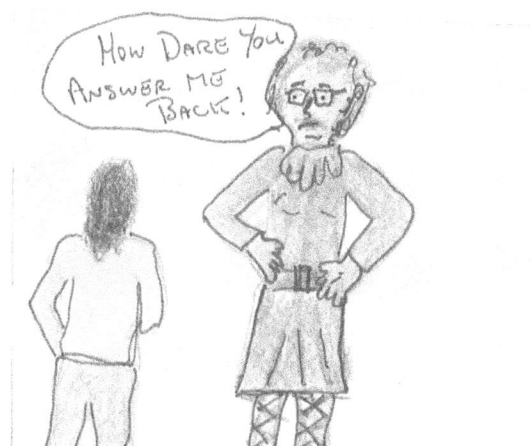

Passive people tend to believe all criticisms that they receive.	Aggressive people try to punish us for daring to criticise them.

BEHAVIOUR TYPES AND CRITICISM.

How do different behaviour types respond to criticism?

- Passive people will tend to take the criticism on board, internalising it and believe it to be completely true. "I expect that they are right, I must be a complete idiot".

- Aggressive people will act defensively coming back with a return criticism, "Who do you think you're calling an idiot? I bet you couldn't do it any better, I bet you couldn't even do it at all!"

- Indirectly aggressive people will try to play on our emotions making us feel guilty for daring to criticise them. They will probably say nothing, but will just go off and sulk.

Any improvement upon these approaches has to be worth a try, so let's see how an assertive person handles criticism.

Now do Exercise 90.

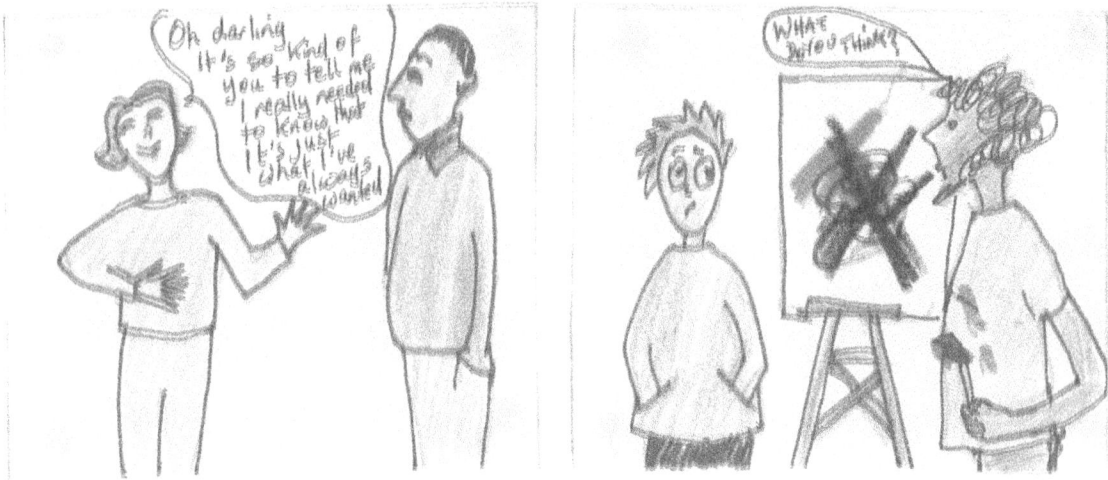

We need to view criticism as a useful gift.		**We need feedback from others to help us to make decisions.**

RECEIVING CRITICISM ASSERTIVELY.

We need to change the way that we currently view criticism. Imagine that you have decided to invest a lot of money setting up your own business as a furniture maker. Unfortunately, although you think that your standard of work is very good because your mother said that she likes it, the reality is that it is terrible. None of your friends have the heart to tell you that because they know how much criticism upsets you. Would you prefer to invest in a business that will soon go bust or would you prefer to receive some honest feedback about the standard of your work?

The reality is that without criticism (or honest negative feedback) these are the types of mistakes that we could very easily make. Every decision that we ever make is based upon previous feedback that we have received. In order to reach any decision we always have to weigh up the positive against the negative, if we do not have any negative information upon which to base our decision, it becomes impossible to be objective. In such circumstances, setting up a furniture making business would seem like a good idea, because all of the feedback received to date would have been only positive feedback.

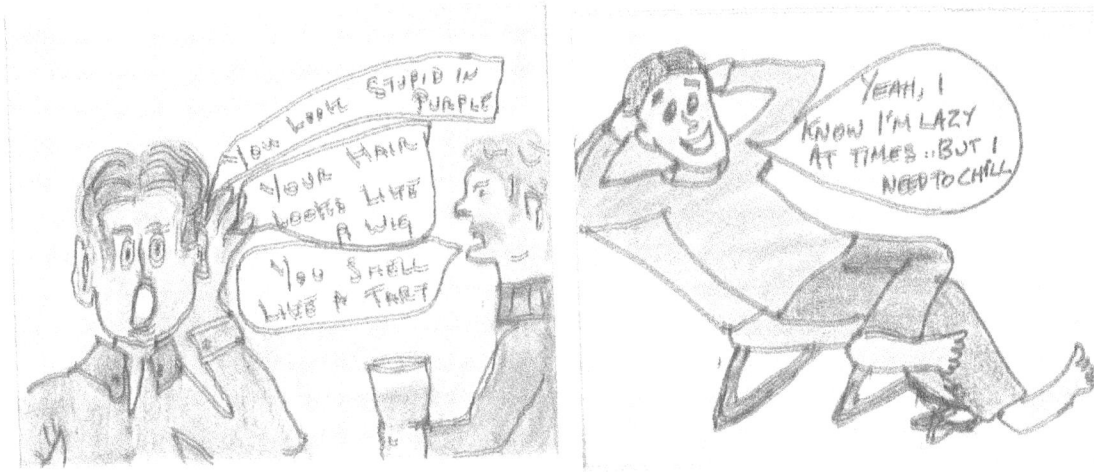

Learn to listen carefully to criticisms.		Identify if they have any validity or are they invalid put-downs.

DEALING WITH CRITICISM ASSERTIVELY.

We have now established that we need criticism in order to make balanced and informed decisions. That however, does not mean that all criticisms are valid. Some will be completely true, some partly true, some wholly untrue and some malicious put-downs. So we need to establish a filtering process so that we can take in the worthwhile information and reject all the unhelpful rubbish without allowing any of it to stick.

STEP 1: Learn to listen to the criticism constructively without jumping to any immediate conclusions. What are they actually saying? Do you understand what they are saying? If not ask for more information and specific examples.

STEP 2: Do you think that the criticism is true, partly true, wholly untrue, or a put-down? Sometimes we need to do a lot of soul searching, we might want to find out what other people think, do they see us in the same light? Have people criticised us for this in the past? Is it something that we always deny because we find it too painful to deal with?

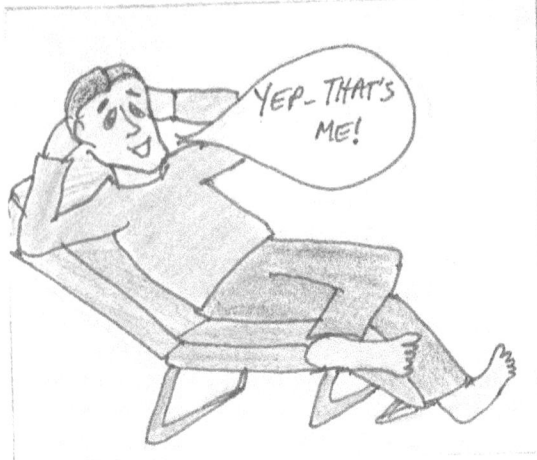

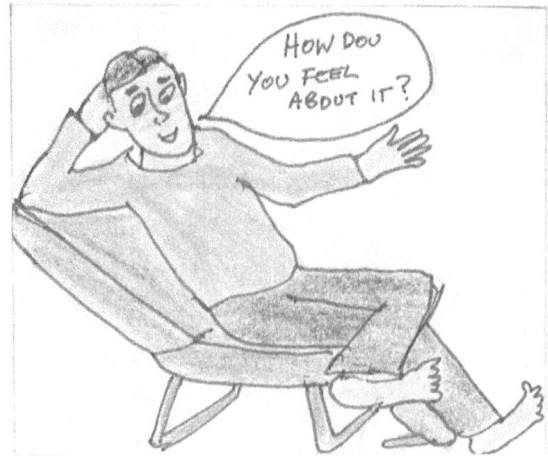

If you are criticised about something that is true, agree with it.	Find out how the thing that you are being criticised for affects others.

HANDLING CRITICISM ASSERTIVELY.

STEP 3: If the criticism is true, agree with it. Why should somebody telling us something about ourselves that we already know and accept cause us any pain? We may also wish to add a statement about how we feel about it along with an enquiry as to how it affects them.

EXAMPLE: "Yes I am very untidy but it doesn't really bother me, how does it affect you?"

See how we have now reversed the situation. They now have to either deny that our untidiness causes them any problem, which would mean that they had no reason to mention it in the first place, or they are forced to tell us the exact effect that our untidiness has on them. This will then help us all to work out an amicable solution.

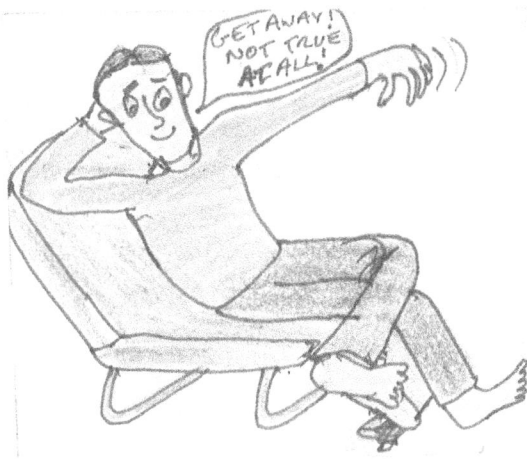

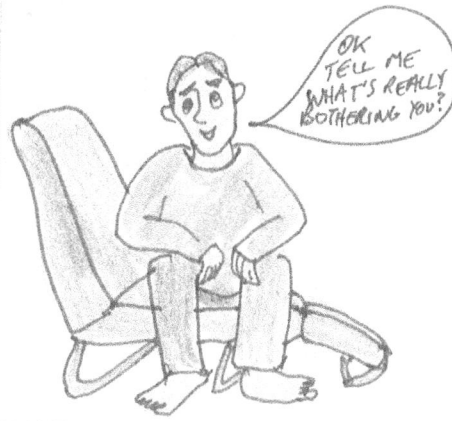

Reject criticisms that are not true.		Encourage others to say what they really need to.

DISCOVER WHY THEY REALLY WANT TO CRITICISE YOU.

STEP 4: If the criticism is partly true, we need to agree with the valid part of it but reject the invalid part. Then we need to enquire why they have come to this judgement of us. Then finally ask how it affects them.

EXAMPLE: **"Yes I am afraid that I am sometimes late, but I do not agree that I am always late. What is it that makes you think that?"**

They are now forced to tell you why they think that you are always late, which gives you a chance to study the evidence and if possible rectify the situation. You can now add your enquiry. "I see, so it is mainly when I am late on a Thursday that I cause you a problem, why exactly is that?"

See how we have helped them to tell us exactly what it is that they need to say to us. Assertive communication also involves encouraging and helping others to be more open and honest about their true feelings as well. By using this approach we have successfully avoided any ill feeling or conflict that could so easily have arisen out of such a delicate situation.

Now do Exercise 91.

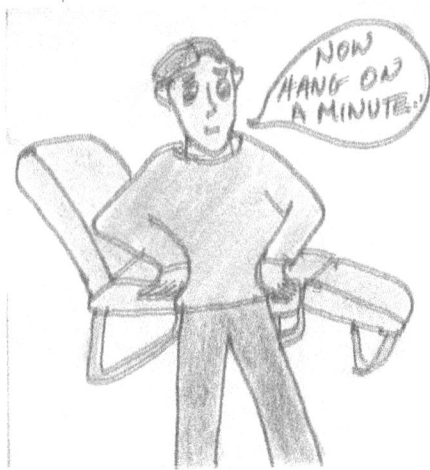

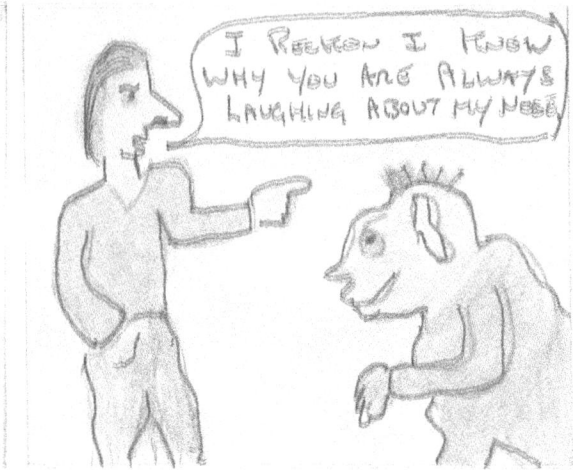

Learn how to challenge and reject untrue criticisms.	Expose the true intent and meaning behind any put-downs.

UNTRUE CRITICISMS AND PUT-DOWNS.

STEP 5: If a criticism is untrue, we need to clearly reject it, add a personal affirmation, disclose our true feelings about what they have just said and add an enquiry as to why they believe this to be true.

"I disagree, I think that I am very good at my job and I feel hurt by what you have just said. What makes you think that I am a useless mechanic?"

Again you have been able to project your true emotions and they have been given a chance to tell you exactly how they have reached their decision. Now you both have an opportunity to rectify the situation.

STEP 6: Put-downs are subtly malicious personal attacks that often use sarcasm or humour to put across powerful and damning messages. We need to directly challenge put-downs so that we can expose the true intent behind the remark. We can challenge put-downs by firstly disclosing how they have just made us feel. "I feel very offended by what you have just said". Then we can ask them to clarify what they actually mean. "I'm confused by what you just said, could you explain in more detail?" Finally we need to end on a positive personal statement. "Yes I am a good mechanic, I think the fact that I am a woman is irrelevant.

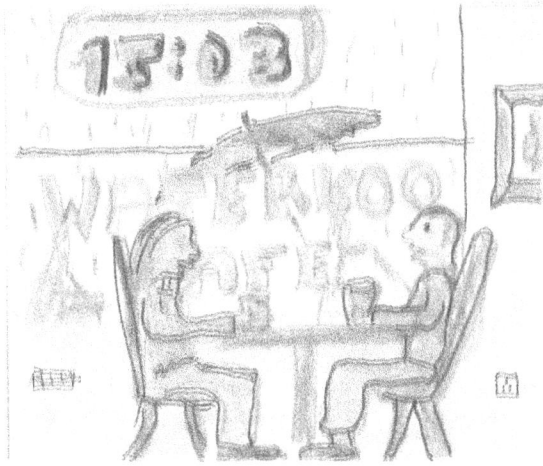

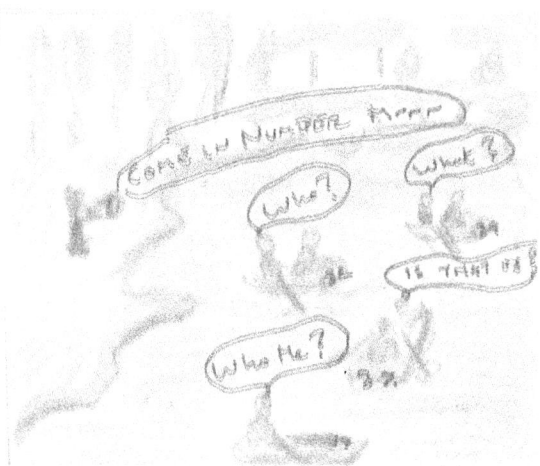

Do not get over-emotional pick the time and the place.	**Be specific and clear, express how it affects you.**

HOW TO CRITICSE OTHER PEOPLE.

Now that we have learnt how to deal with being criticised, we need to learn how to give criticism to others so that they can benefit from our feedback as well. How do you currently give out criticism? If you are a passive person, you might avoid it altogether. If you are an aggressive person you will probably just try to manipulate people to change, rather than explain the meaning behind your actions. These responses all seem far from ideal. So let's see how to criticise assertively.

STEP 1: Check what you really want to say, avoid getting worked up or over emotional.

STEP 2: Choose the right time and place, do not criticise in front of other people.

STEP 3: Avoid personalising the criticism. Make it non-judgemental, use examples.

STEP 4: Express your own feelings, the effect that the behaviour is having upon you.

STEP 5: Get them to express their point of view and make sure that you listen.

STEP 6: Work towards a compromise or resolution.

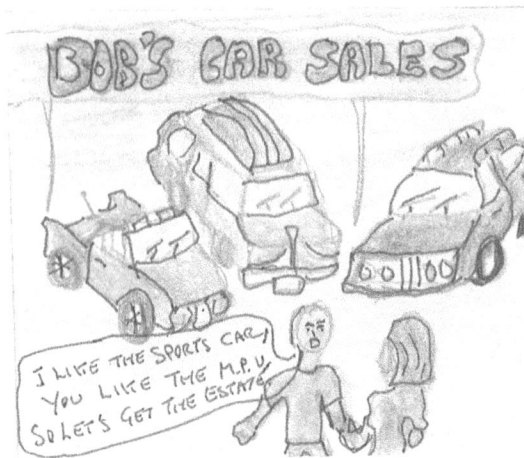

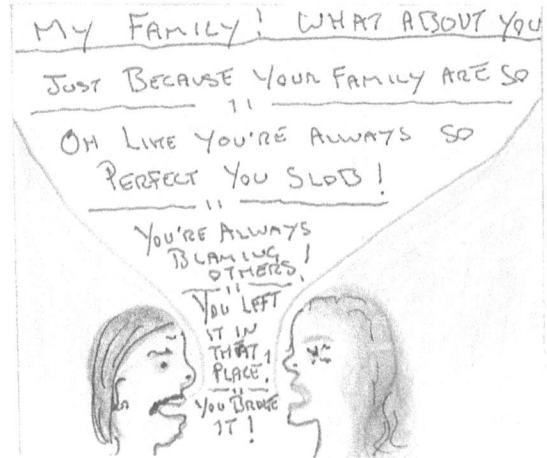

Always work towards a point of agreement.	Do not allow disagreements to expand outwards.

DIRECT THE CONFRONTATION BACK TO ITS CAUSE.

Notice how that instead of getting angry and defensive, we have used being criticised to help the other person say what they really wanted to say to us all along. If we can imagine an equilateral triangle, in most disagreements we start off with one trigger (the top angle). The argument then expands and all the disagreements and irritations from previous occasions get brought into the argument. Eventually this flat line at the bottom is reached, with both parties stood in different corners, a long way apart from each other.

With assertive communication the idea is to work from two different corners towards the top angle, so that we have pinpointed and dealt with the cause of the disagreement directly.

Now do Exercise 92.

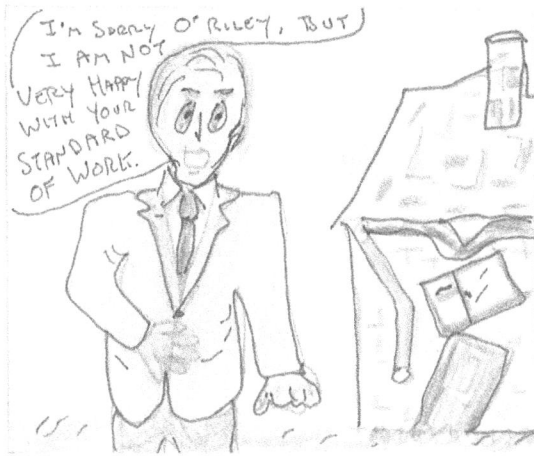

| Giving out criticism can feel very uncomfortable. | Try to focus on the positive reasons for criticising. |

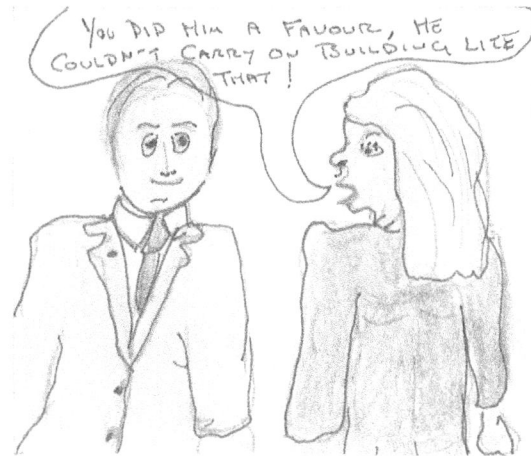

CRITICISING OTHERS IS NEVER EASY.

Even when you follow steps 1-6, giving criticism can still feel very uncomfortable. This is usually because we are so aware of how painful receiving criticism has been for us in the past that we do not want to put anyone else through the same discomfort. Yet if we fail to give constructive criticism, we could be setting somebody up for more hurt in the long run. The longer we put off giving the criticism, the longer we prolong the agony.

We are far more likely to give constructive criticism if we deal with a situation assertively as soon as it arises, rather than allowing emotions to build up. Nobody can tell you exactly when you should or should not criticise, it is down to you to judge the situation for yourself.

Now do Exercise 93.

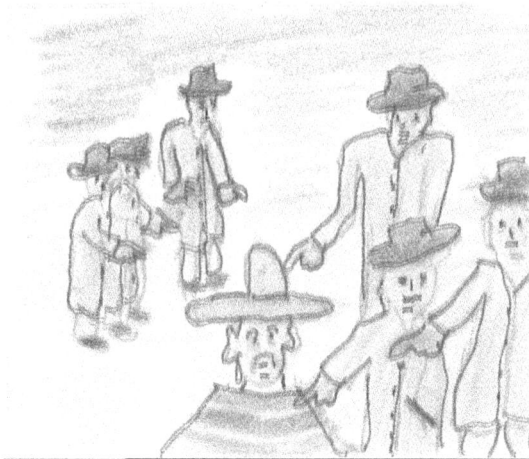

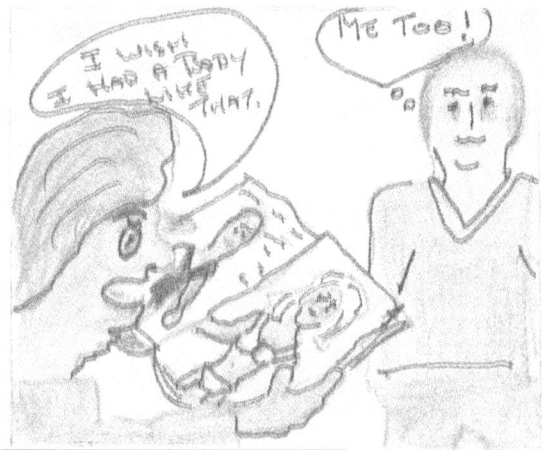

We are made to feel like an outcast if we do not conform to society's "norms".	"Women should always look stunningly attractive".

SOCIETY'S MESSAGES ABOUT OUR SEXUALITY.

It is important to be aware of the messages that society and the media project on us and recognise the effect they have on the roles we assume in our lives. Assertiveness is about believing in ourselves, following our own thoughts and feelings and not being afraid to express our individuality. Society's messages tend to all be about conforming to stereotypes that the media have created. Some of these images revolve around money and glamour - this has the effect of making us feel bad about ourselves if we are unable to obtain them. Think about the effect that some of these statements have had upon you.

- Men need to be tough.

- Men should not be emotional.

- Men should be excellent providers.

- Women should always look attractive.

Now do Exercise 93.

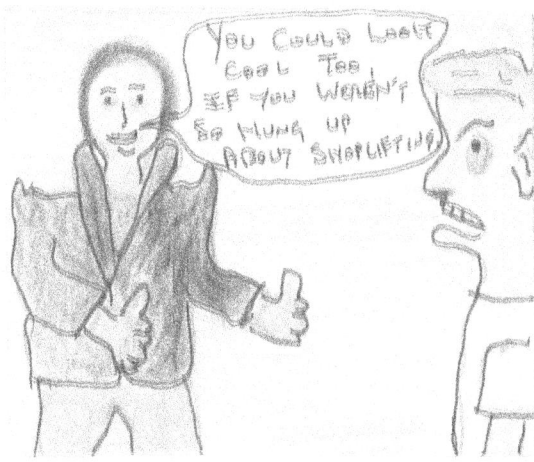

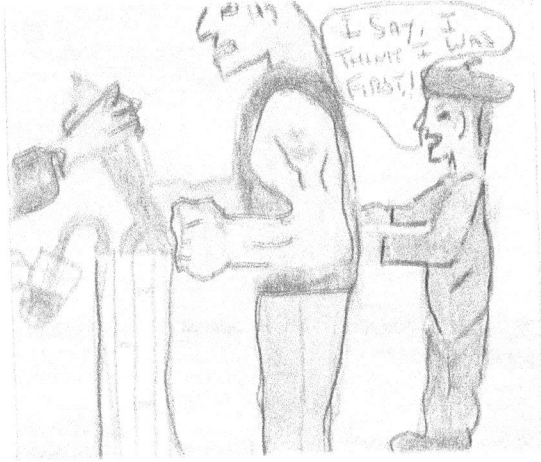

Do not allow others to push you into behaving like them.	You will not always achieve perfect assertive behaviour.

THE POWER OF POSSESSING ASSERTIVENESS.

Assertiveness is all about being in control of ourselves and having a feeling of personal power one thing that we have to constantly be aware of is the effect that others will have upon us. Passive people will hand over power to us, which will tempt us to behave in a directly aggressive manner. Directly aggressive people will try to abuse our power, which may make us feel like giving up and behaving passively. Indirectly aggressive people will misuse their own power, which will tempt us to behave likewise in order to compete with them. So being assertive and keeping on track is an ongoing process that we need to continuously work at.

You will have failures, we all do, but as long as you can see and understand how the failures happened, what you have done and learn from them, then you have the power to be an assertive person.

Now do Exercise 94.

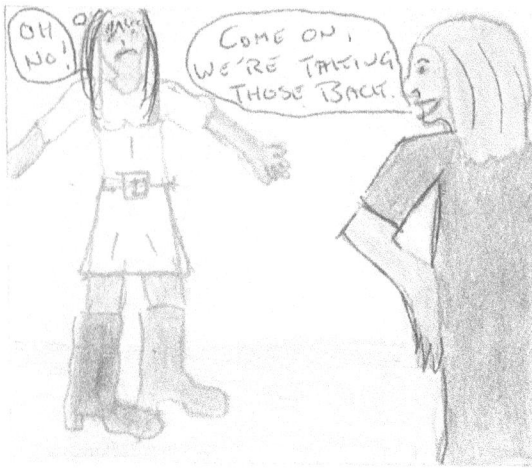

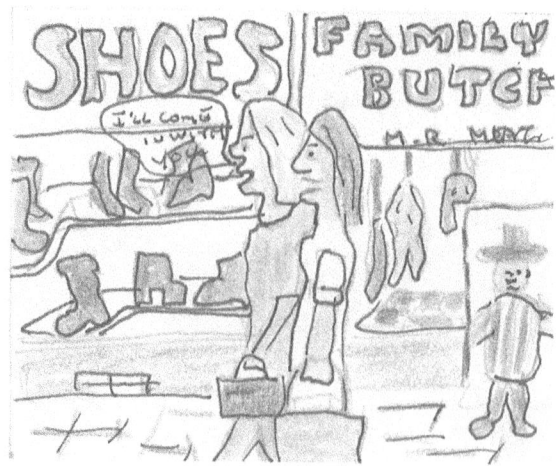

| Encourage them to develop their assertiveness skills. | Support them when they struggle to get it right. |

WHAT CAN FAMILY AND FRIENDS DO TO HELP?

It is not easy to become assertive, especially when you have spent many years developing your own behaviour patterns in order to survive. Anybody making the effort to change needs all of the encouragement and support that they can get. Try not to be cynical or derogatory about their new style of behaviour. Read through the information about behaviour types and body language so that you can identify when they are being assertive, aggressive or passive. Give them honest positive feedback about their performance. Respect their rights. When they want to work towards a compromise, try to be as helpful and obliging as possible. If they are failing to be clear, point this out to them. Give them feedback about the messages you are getting from their body language. Tell them when they are failing to acknowledge your rights.

Remember that a lot of people who have been passive tend to swing into being fairly aggressive when they first try to be assertive, so make allowances for this. Most importantly, be there for them when they feel that they might have failed.

DEPRESSION

DRUGS AND ALCOHOL

ANXIETY

ANGER

ASSERTIVENESS

STRESS

LOW SELF-ESTEEM

It is easier to control the
raging force of a volcano
if you have already taken
the correct precautions.

If you wait and do nothing
until it erupts,
the consequences can be
completely devastating.

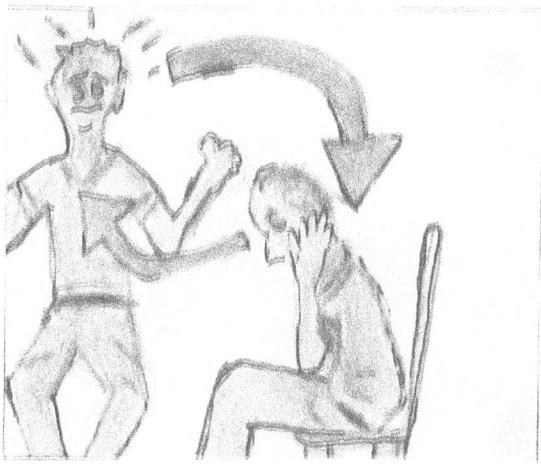

Anger and depression can fuel each other	**Understand how your own anger patterns work so that you can override them.**

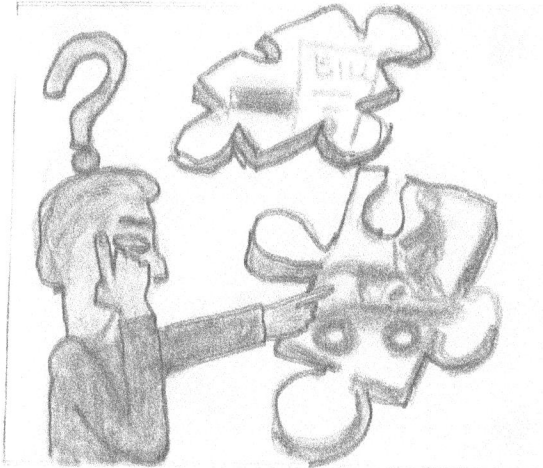

THE LINK BETWEEN ANGER AND DEPRESSION.

There is a strong link between our feelings of anger and our depression; both are capable of fuelling each other. If we constantly lose control of our temper we will start hurting the people around us who really matter. Eventually we will push them away and destroy our relationship with them leaving us feeling sad, lonely and guilty. We also run the risk of getting into trouble and breaking the law, this can lead to us losing our jobs or possibly even our freedom and so we will become depressed.

If we are depressed we run the risk of getting very angry as we become more and more frustrated and angry about our own predicament. We may also be plagued by unpleasant past life events, which can make us feel both sad and angry. If we take the time to discover and understand how our anger patterns really work, we can start to develop an awareness and an insight that will help us to override this primitive response and allow us to function on a more intellectual plane.

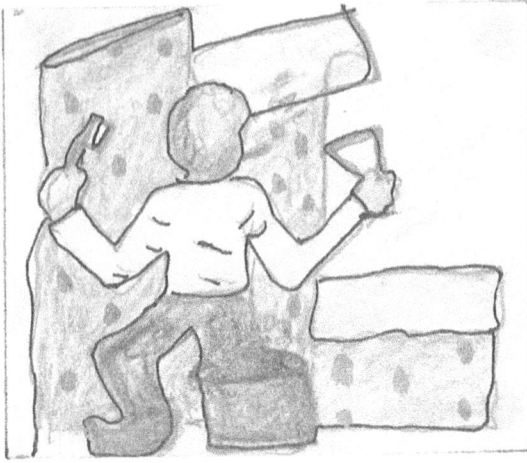

It is a natural emotion that occurs when we feel overwhelmed.	Everyone has to find a way to deal with their anger.

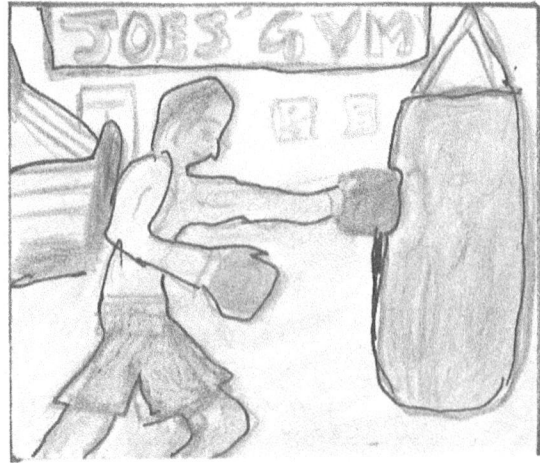

WHAT IS ANGER?

Anger is a natural emotion, no different or worse than any other emotion. It tends to happen when we reach a point of feeling unable to cope, either due to a lack of coping skills, inappropriate learnt behaviour or overwhelming feelings of frustration. Anger is generally considered to be a primitive response because we allow it to override our higher intellectual brain function.

In primitive times it was a good response because it supplied us with the brute force needed to tackle frustrating situations. Today however, very few problems can be tackled with sheer brute force and poor thinking ability, so we view anger as a very bad destructive emotion. We tend to try and ignore its existence, passing it off as somebody else's problem when in reality it affects every one of us. Even people who never get angry have a problem with anger because they are failing to deal with their true emotions. If an emotion is blocked off it will eventually come out disguised as another emotion such as depression.

Now do Exercise 95.

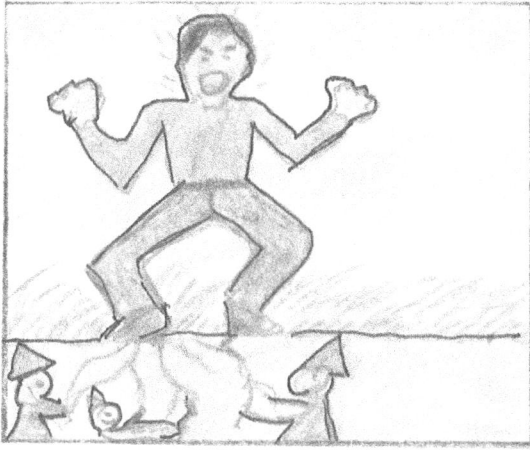

It is the root cause of our anger that we need to explore.	We may need to change our own perspective on past events.

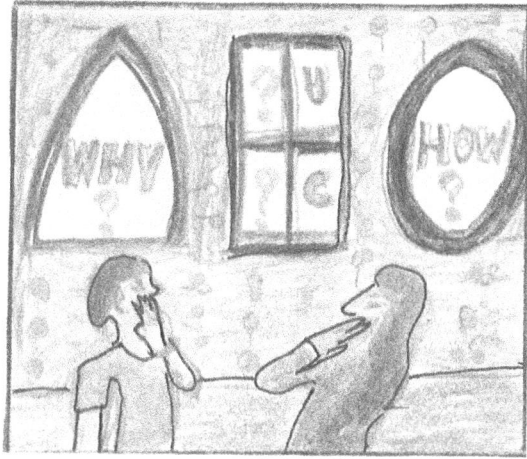

SOME REASONS FOR FEELING ANGRY.

There are many reasons why we might feel angry or irritated, but when we are suffering from prolonged feelings of anger, the causes tend to originate from one of the following:

- Feeling victimised.

- Feeling that life has been very unfair.

- Missing out on opportunities.

- Never having any opportunities.

- Suffering from a long-term illness or disability.

- Unresolved childhood issues.

- Always being a very passive person.

- Being raised by parents with anger management problems.

- Being a victim of abuse or inequality.

- Feeling frustrated by our own shortcomings.

Now do Exercise 96.

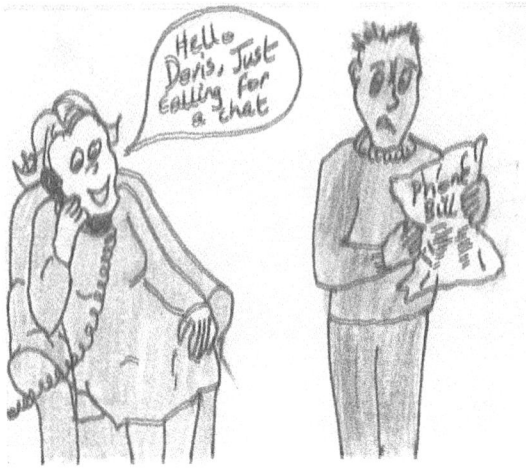

There is always something to get angry about.		We have to learn to view things in a new light.

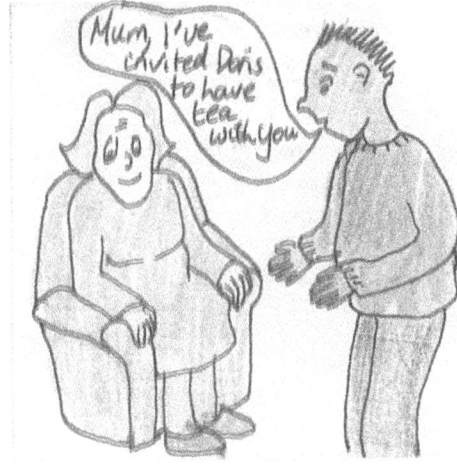

WHY GET ANGRY?

It is not difficult to find something to get angry about if we want to. We are constantly being bombarded with frustrating triggers such as gridlock on our roads, financial worries, technological advances, job insecurity, the list is endless. These problems are not going to go away so we have to learn to deal with them appropriately.

If the problems are not going to change and getting angry about the problems isn't going to improve anything either, how can we appropriately deal with these problems? The only two things that we have the power to change are our own perspective and the way that we deal with our initial feelings of frustration. If we can gain some control over these, then we can also gain some control over our anger.

Now do Exercise 97.

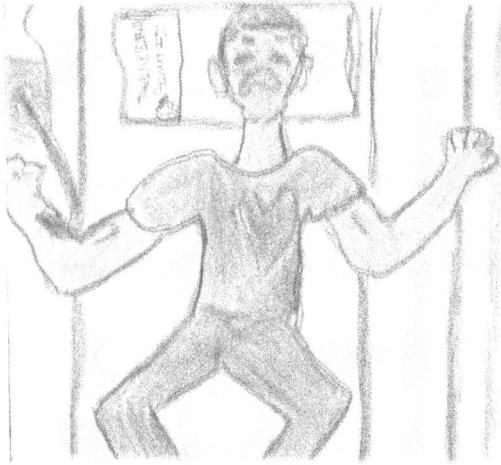

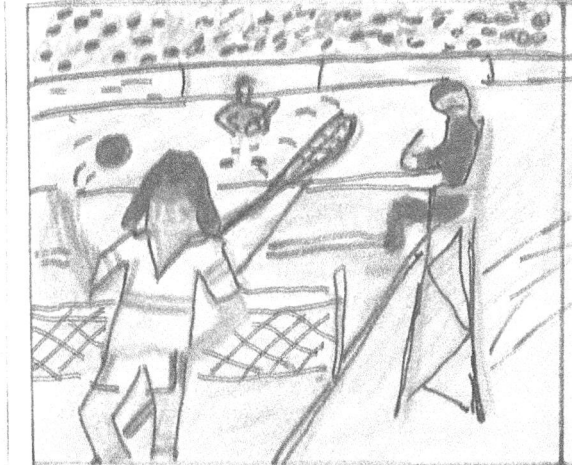

| Anger weakens our hearts. | It causes major behavioural problems. |

THE PRICE THAT WE PAY FOR GETTING ANGRY.

There are many problems associated with constantly getting angry.

- Firstly, it is not good for our health. It puts an incredible strain on our hearts, decreasing their pumping efficiency and increasing our chances of suffering a stroke or heart attack.

- Secondly, it has a terrible effect upon our behaviour, making us loud, threatening and abusive. Sometimes we can resort to smashing things up or becoming violent. People start to avoid us because they think of us as unstable and dangerous.

- Thirdly, we feel ashamed of ourselves for losing control and saying things that we wished we hadn't. If we acted violently, we might be overwhelmed with guilt, throwing us into feelings of despair and deep depression. We might also end up on the wrong side of the law, which could lead to a criminal conviction and the possibility of losing our job, our home, or possibly our loved ones.

Now do Exercise 98.

147

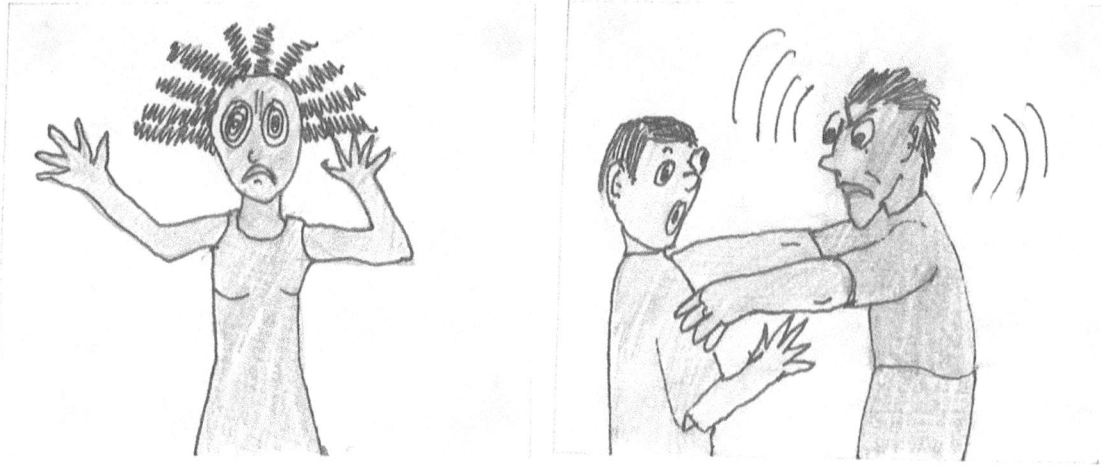

When we go into rage our brain stops working.	Never try to reason with someone who is in a state of rage.

WHEN ANGER TURNS TO RAGE.

When people talk about seeing red, they are talking about a feeling of extreme anger and a loss of control known as rage. When we are in this state, our brain has become so overwhelmed that it is now no longer able to reason or decipher information appropriately. Rage is a very dangerous state to be in because we are quite literally capable of murder! We are out of control and extremely dangerous!

It is impossible to reason with somebody who is in a state of rage, they are best left alone in a safe environment to gradually calm down. This approach could be referred to as "damage limitation". No amount of talking to them will have any effect because they will be unable to take anything in. Some people come out of their rage state unable to recall anything that they have just done.

The best way to avoid this dangerous state is to learn how to deal with your feelings of anger appropriately before you allow yourself to reach a state of rage.

Now do Exercise 99.

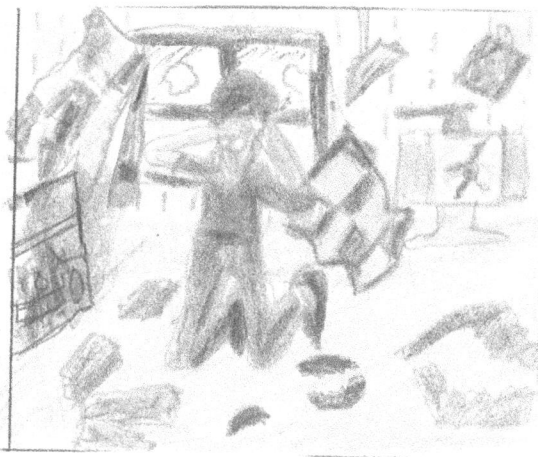

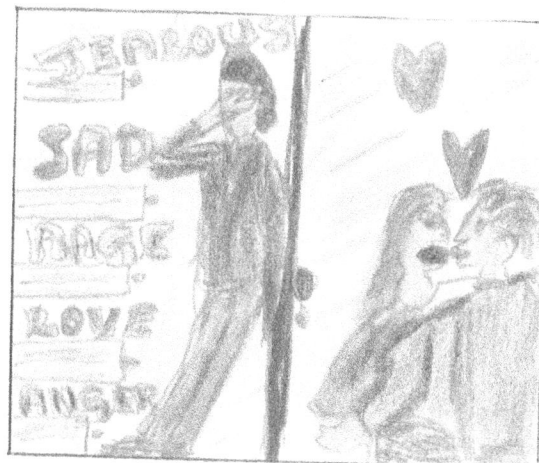

| We can fall into depression when we realise what we have done. | If we start to fear our own anger we can start to hide our true emotions. |

THE AFTER-EFFECTS OF RAGE BEHAVIOUR.

After experiencing an episode of severe rage most of us will fall into a state of despair and depression. This is because we feel deeply ashamed of ourselves for how we have just behaved and we feel sad that we have hurt others around us. We also develop a fear of ourselves. If we can lose control once, we can lose control again. What might we be capable of doing the next time that it happens? Will we be able to control it? Can we repair the damage that we have just done to people around us?

If we start to fear our own temper, we can develop poor coping strategies such as denying our own feelings and emotions, bottling them up and failing to express them, becoming inward and reserved. Yes, these are the exact same behaviour traits that lead to depression.

Now do Exercise 100.

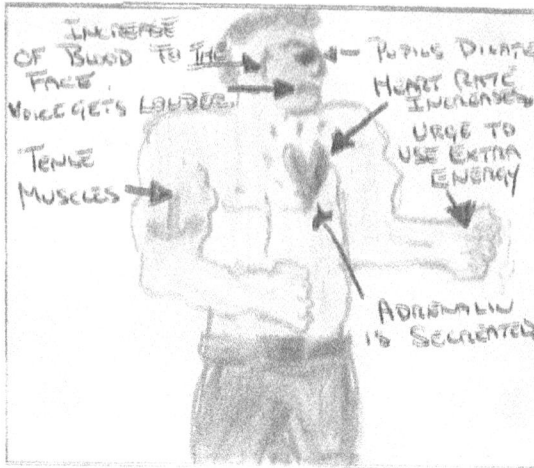

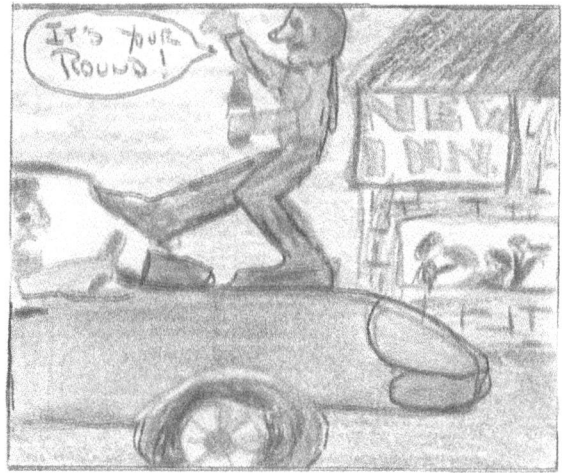

| Identify the changes that start to occur in your body when you feel angry. | How do you think and behave? |

HOW ANGER AFFECTS US.

How do we know when we are about to get angry? What physical sensations do we start to get in our bodies? What thoughts take over our minds? How do we start to behave? Are there any particular places, people, or situations that seem to trigger off our anger? These are the key questions that we need to answer for ourselves in order to be able to identify when we are about to become angry. It is only when we can identify the feelings leading up to anger that we can start to gain some control of ourselves. If we can learn to control and deal with these feelings of anger before they control us, we will have the power to control our own anger.

Now do Exercise 100.

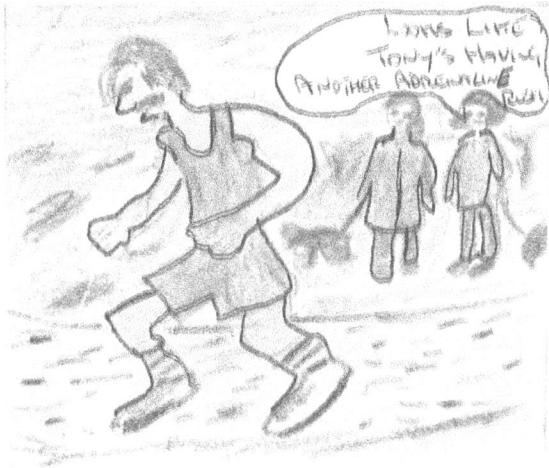

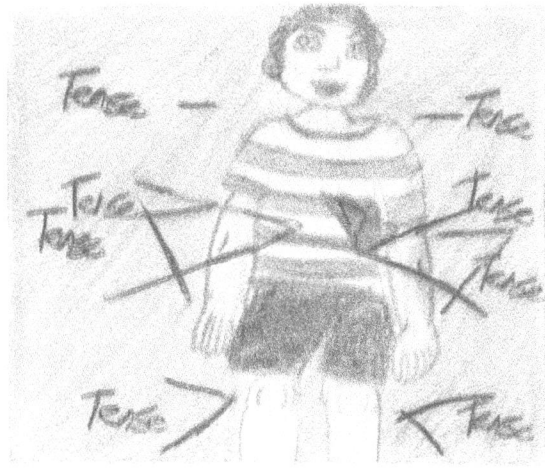

When adrenaline is released we experience an energy rush.	Usual reactions include tense muscles and a racing heart.

RECOGNISE YOUR PHYSICAL REPSONSES TO ANGER.

The usual physical reactions we tend to experience when anger builds up include:

- Tense muscles.

- Heavy breathing.

- Increased heart rate.

- Increased sweating.

- Dilated pupils.

- Increased feelings of strength and energy.

This is all due to the release of extra adrenaline. As with anxiety, blood is diverted away from non-essential organs and so our ability to think reasonably and rationally becomes severely affected. Have you ever noticed how difficult it is to string a sentence together when you are angry? This is why we use short messages such as," I'll kill you". "You've had it". Our brains cannot cope with complex messages when we are feeling angry.

Now do Exercises 101 & 102.

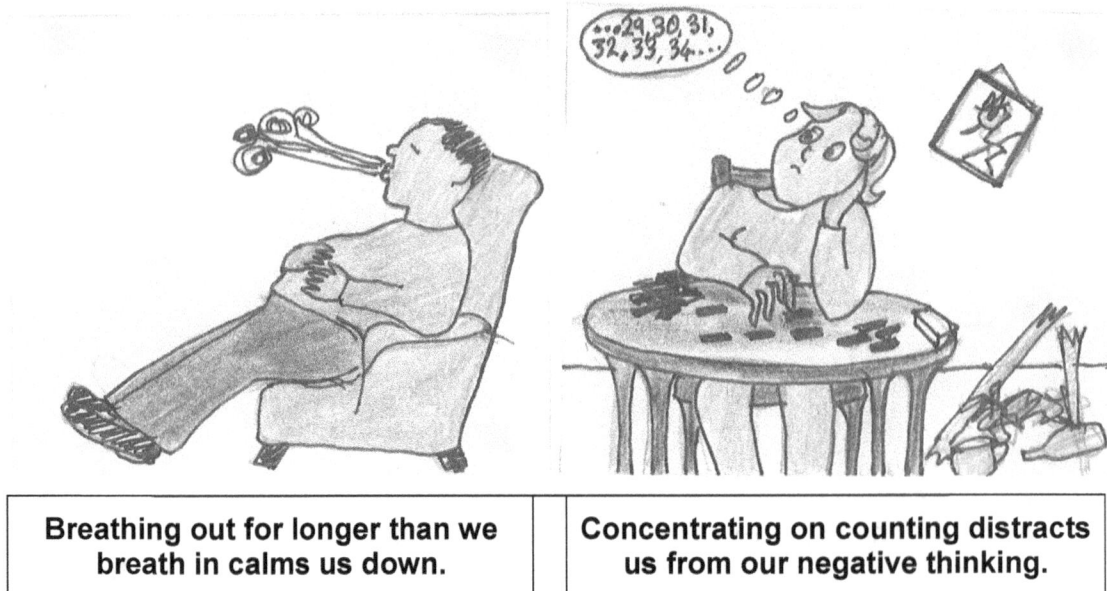

| Breathing out for longer than we breath in calms us down. | Concentrating on counting distracts us from our negative thinking. |

A QUICK RELAXATION TECHNIQUE FOR RELIEVING THE PHYSICAL RESPONSES TO ANGER.

In order to reverse the over-stimulation of the sympathetic nervous system which gives rise to all of the increased agitation that we feel, we need to try this basic relaxation technique.

1. Inhale to the count of 4.

2. Exhale to the count of 6.

3. Wait for the count of 4.

4. Begin the cycle again.

This technique works by stimulating the parasympathetic nervous system; this system is a far calmer one which triggers a relaxation response. Thereby making it impossible to become over-agitated and angry.   By concentrating on this counting, we also distract our thought processes away from the anger trigger.

Now do Exercise 103.

152

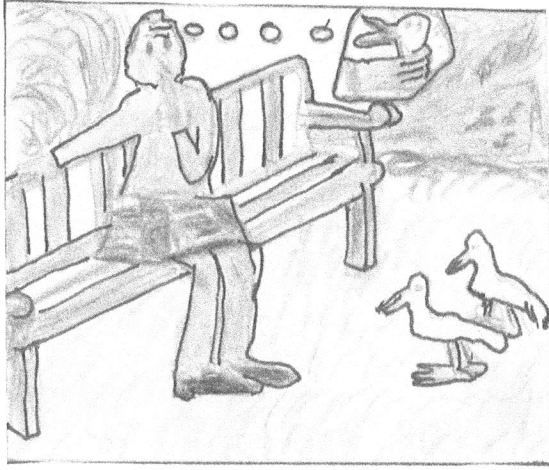

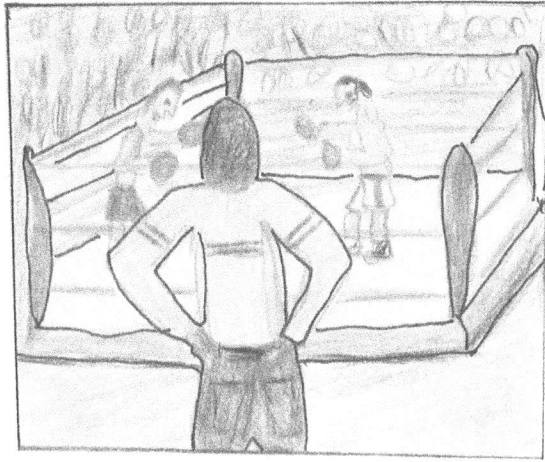

Allow yourself some thinking time. Why am I reacting like this?	**View the situation from a neutral perspective, what would be the best possible outcome.**

CHALLENGING OUR ANGRY THOUGHTS.

It is very easy for us to let angry thoughts totally take over. Think how quickly we can become angry with other motorists when we feel that they are taking advantage of us. If we allow ourselves time to stop and think we can probably recall instances when we have behaved in a similar manner due to being lost or in a hurry. It is important to always allow ourselves some thinking time.

- What is the angry thought?

- Who is it directed at?

- Why am I reacting like this? Am I in imminent danger?

- What outcome do I really want from this situation?

Try and view the situation as if you were totally removed from it. If this was Mr A and Mr B what would be the best possible outcome? How could they resolve this in a mature civilised manner?

Now do Exercise 104.

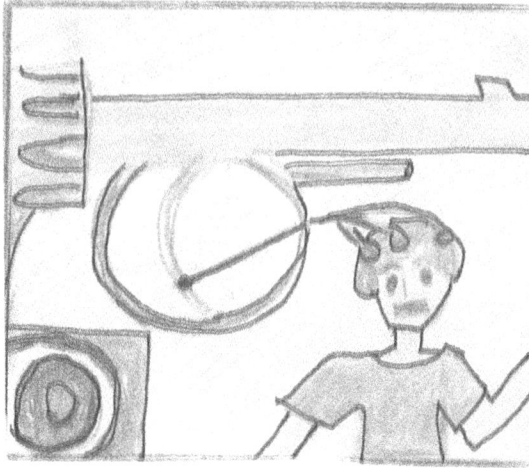

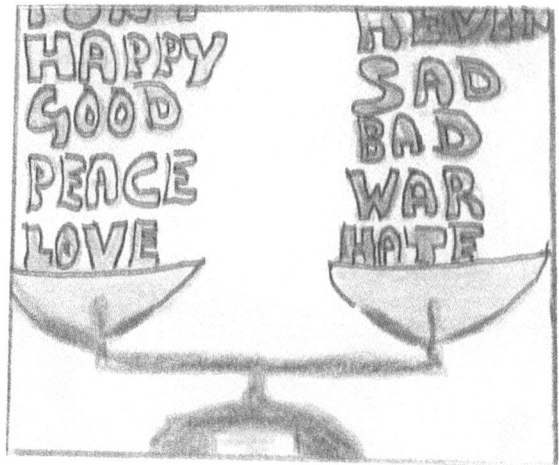

| Anger can be triggered by the way that we think. | Try to adopt a more balanced view to your thinking patterns. |

COMMON THINKING ERRORS THAT FUEL ANGER.

If we find ourselves frequently getting angry, we are most probably using a lot of thinking errors. We may be taking things too personally and so find ourselves feeling hurt and resentful. We may be constantly looking for and expecting others to criticise us. We may be focusing our thinking on negative events and ignoring all of the positive ones.

If we are perfectionists, we may find that we are expecting too much from ourselves, as well as others around us. If we adopt an aggressive or a passive style of personality, we may find that we create and fuel anger in others. If we think in all or nothing terms, the frequent disappointments that we are bound to experience will make us very angry. We may also need to re-examine and challenge some of our beliefs that seemed right in the past but now tend to cause us difficulties.

Now do Exercise 105.

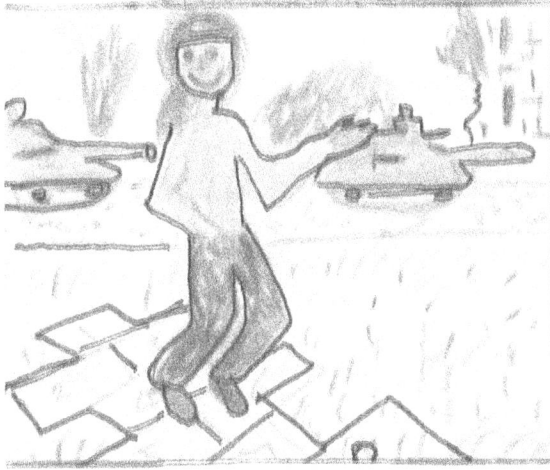

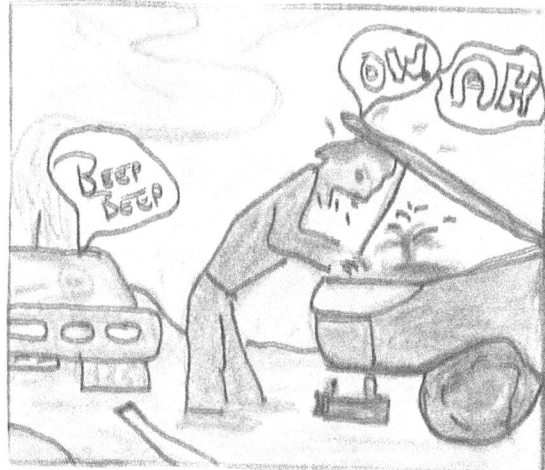

| Our mood determines how we react to things. | We are far more likely to get angry if we are in a bad mood already. |

OUR MOOD DETERMINES OUR LEVEL OF ANGER.

Imagine that you are walking along a beautiful sandy beach on a hot day with an ice cream in your hand. You are pleased to be on holiday, happy to be surrounded by family and friends and you are looking forward to going surfing. Suddenly a soft beach ball hits you on the back of the head. How do you respond?

You are walking along the same beach on the same day with the same people, but this time you are concerned about money. The cash point machine just rejected your card, you had to borrow some money from your friend to pay for your ice cream, and you were looking forward to doing some surfing in the sea but now the waves have died down. You think about how useless your job is because it doesn't pay you enough money to survive on. Then a soft beach ball hits you on the head. How do you respond?

See how the situation is exactly the same but our mood is completely different. Mood is our strongest indicator when it comes to predicting the likelihood of us losing our temper.

Now do Exercise 106.

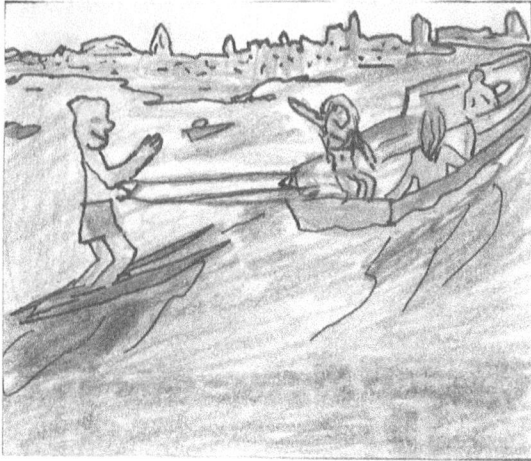

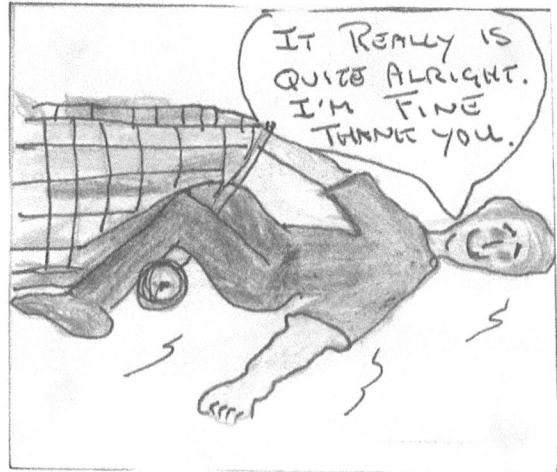

| We need to make some positive changes to our lives if we want to change our low mood. | If we can gain some control over our mood, we can gain some control over our anger. |

CONTROL YOUR MOOD BY TAKING POSITIVE ACTION.

If we are constantly in a bad mood it is a sure sign that we are not very happy with certain aspects of our lives. We therefore have two choices; (a) either make positive plans to change those aspects of our lives that are making us feel so miserable or (b) change the way that we view them. If we fail to act upon the messages that our bodies are clearly giving us then we run the risk of becoming chronically depressed. If we feel under a lot of pressure we need to balance our lives out by spending more time pursuing pleasurable pursuits. Aerobic sports like running, swimming and cycling not only give us a physical release from pent up energy, they allow us valuable thinking and contemplating time, this can help us to put things into perspective.

When we know that something is going to put us into a bad mood, we can either avoid it, or plan around it in order to minimise its impact upon us. The more control that we gain over our mood, the more control we can gain over our anger.

Now do Exercise 107.

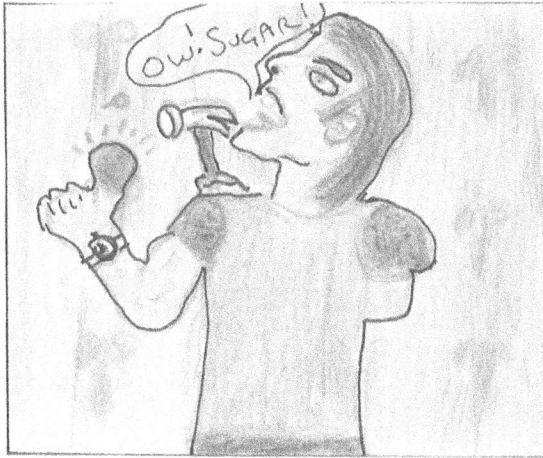

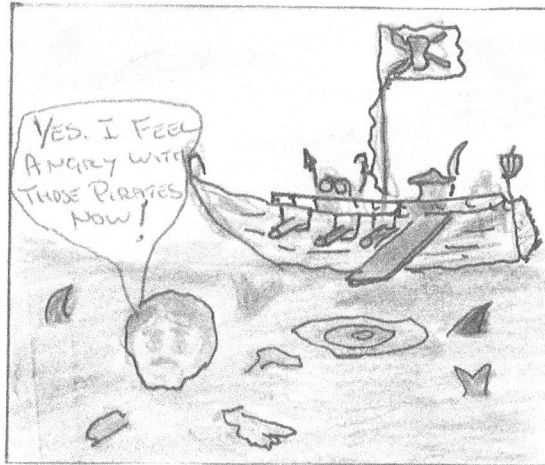

It is natural to feel angry from time to time.	Learn to express the appropriate level of anger to the right person at the right time.

LEARN TO EXPRESS ANGER ASSERTIVELY.

Whatever techniques we use, nothing can take away the fact that from time to time we are still going to experience feelings of anger. We need to accept that this is a natural response and if we deal with it appropriately we should have no need to feel ashamed or guilty about it. Remember we all have a right to feel angry, just as we have a right to feel happy.

If we can learn to express our feelings of anger appropriately to the right person at the right time and at the right level of intensity, we will have no reason to dwell upon past situations because our anger will have been dealt with at the correct time. Sometimes, if we just simply say that we are angry about something it can be sufficient to release the emotion.

We need to always be honest with ourselves about our true emotions so that we can express them appropriately.

Now do Exercise 108.

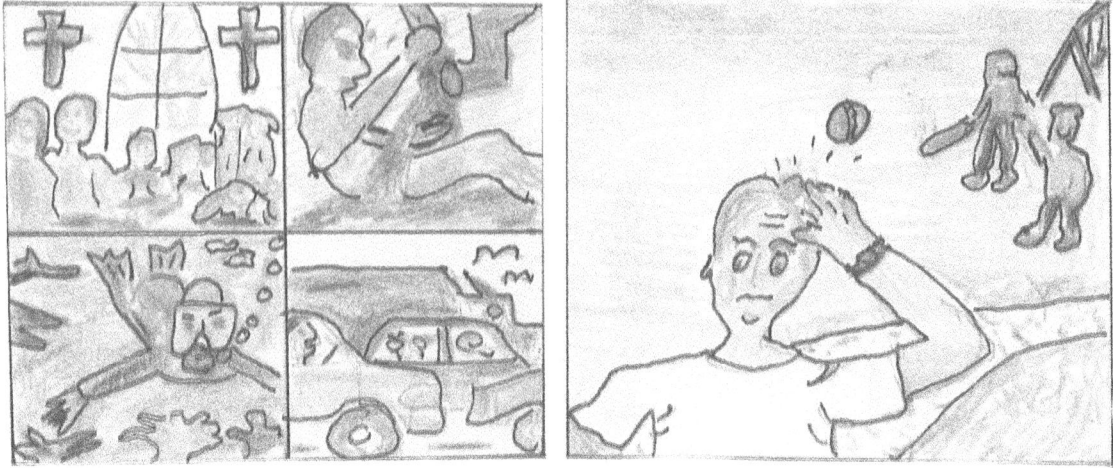

Identify which roles tend to make you susceptible to angry outbursts.	Pinpoint exactly what it is that triggers off your angry response.

RECOGNISE WHICH OF YOUR ROLES CONTAINS THE ANGRY PARTS OF YOUR PERSONALITY.

We all adopt different personality traits depending upon which role we are currently in. Think how different we can be when we are with – a friend, a work colleague, a customer, a cousin, a parent, a volunteer, a partner or a sibling. We are more likely to be prone to anger in some roles than we are in others. If we can identify why certain roles make us prone to anger, then we can start to pinpoint exactly what it is that fuels the anger in us. It may be a certain person that upsets us, or we may even be upset by our own behaviour in these roles.

Understanding exactly what it is that makes us angry increases our chance of gaining some control over it. If we fail to investigate the causes of our anger, we will forever be at the mercy of our own anger patterns.

Now do Exercise 109.

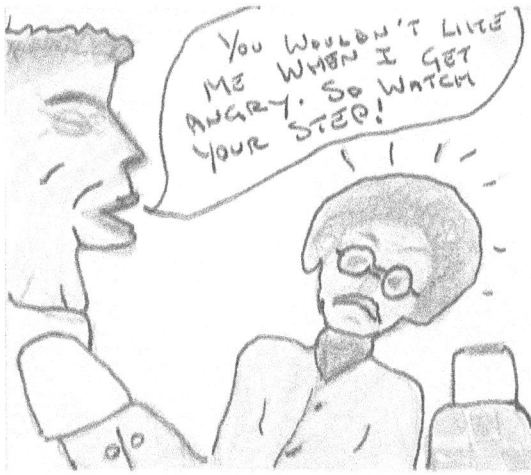

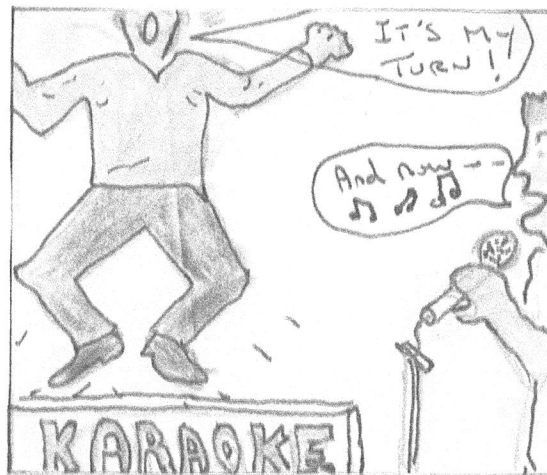

We can sometimes enjoy the power that anger gives us.	We may have to increase the intensity of our anger in order for it to still have any effect.

ARE YOU BENEFITTING FROM YOUR ANGER?

It is common for us to get what we want when we become angry, others tend to fear us, so they do what we want in order to calm the situation down and reduce our anger. We might have learnt to manipulate others by bullying them with our anger. Some of us enjoy the buzz that we get out of the adrenaline rush. A lot of the feelings and sensations of anger are very similar to those that we would experience from an orgasm.

Anger can be used to disguise our own lack of assertiveness. It can give us a feeling of power that we may feel unable to obtain in any other area of our lives. The trouble is that the more frequently we lose our temper, the less effective it becomes because other people become accustomed to it. We now need to reach an even greater degree of anger in order to have any effect and so our anger becomes increasingly worse.

Now do Exercise 110.

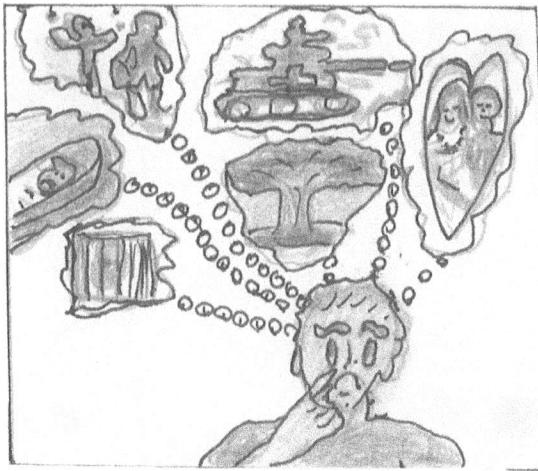

| Are you plagued by past experiences that make you feel angry? | Plan new ways to view these situations, ways that will reduce your anger. |

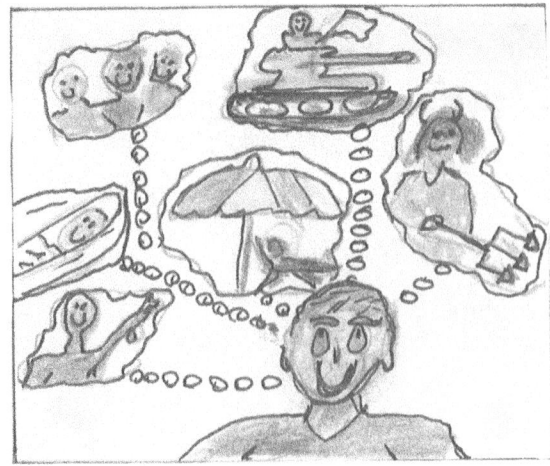

ARE YOU ANGRY ABOUT THE PAST?

we feel constantly angry about something that happened to us a long time ago we need to decide what to do about it now. In some cases it will now be too late for us to return to the situation and change it. Sometimes we can change how we view the situation, we might be able to change our perspective and see the situation differently in a more positive light. We might now be older and wiser and realise that things were not necessarily how we thought they were at the time.

We might now find it easier to forgive and forget. We may choose to work through our thoughts and feelings with a counsellor who will help us to deal with them appropriately. Whatever approach we take, it is important that we realise that getting angry now is not the answer. We need to make a decision today, to change the way that we think about these past issues.

Now do Exercise 111.

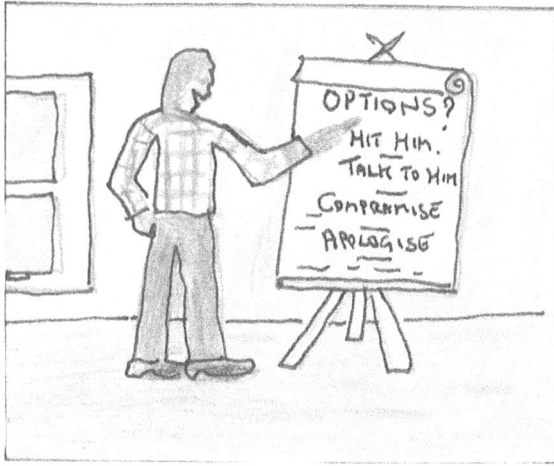

| Effective problem solving can reduce feelings of frustration. | Check that you really have looked at the problem from all angles. |

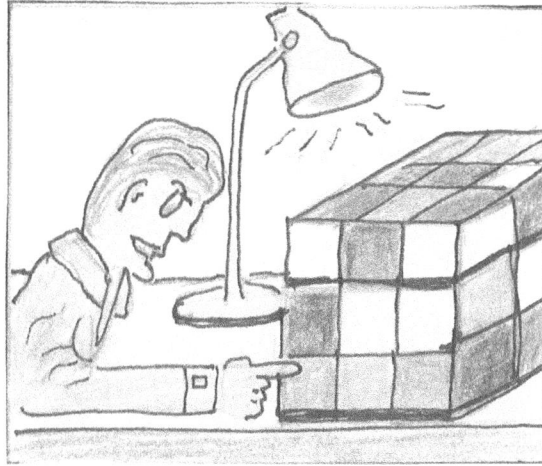

ARE YOU EASILY FRUSTRATED?

We usually feel angry when it seems that we have exhausted all possible options and have failed to produce a positive result. Although this sort of frustration cannot always be avoided, it is worth returning to the "exhausted all options" part before getting angry, because once we get angry we will be unable to effectively problem solve.

- Have you really exhausted all options?

- What would a professional plumber, mechanic, builder, etc., do in this situation?

- Would I benefit by now stopping for a break?

- Would somebody else be able to advise me?

- Am I really a failure if I can't do this?

- Would it be better to employ a professional?

Getting angry and frustrated never produces better workmanship, effective problems solving however does.

Now do Exercise 112.

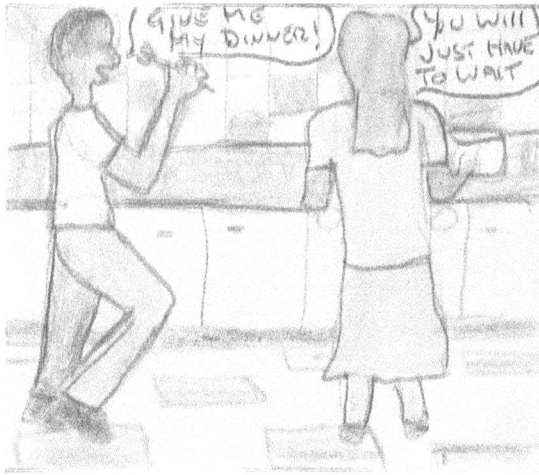

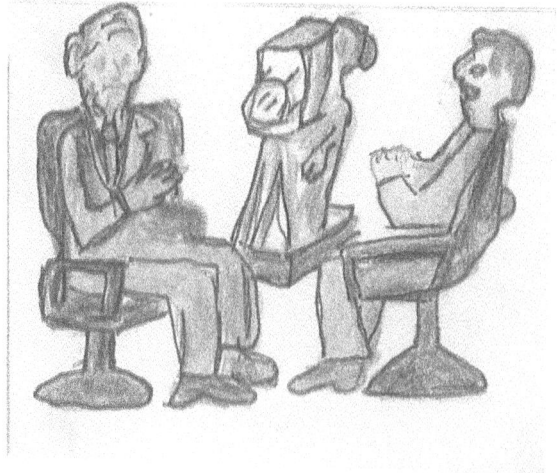

Do not allow angry people to violate your rights or bully you.	Encourage them to talk honestly about their angry feelings.

WHAT CAN FAMILY AND FRIENDS DO TO HELP?

It is very difficult to deal with somebody who is constantly angry so you are going to require a lot of patience and tolerance. Make sure that you do not take the bait, avoid being drawn into their anger and try to avoid arguments, especially when the person is already aroused. Encourage them to express their feelings openly and honestly so that they can discuss the things that make them angry without actually becoming angry. Do not allow yourself to become a victim or an easy target for their anger. Make sure that your rights are not violated by their behaviour. Angry people need to learn that they will not get what they want by bullying you. Point this out clearly to them; encourage them to channel their anger into more constructive pastimes.

Do not allow them to become stuck, explain to them that change is never easy, but it is always possible. Congratulate them on any progress that they make. Show a keen interest in any plans that they make to help them to deal with their anger. Always remain positive and optimistic.

DEPRESSION

ANGER

ANXIETY

DRUGS AND ALCOHOL

ASSERTIVENESS

STRESS

LOW SELF-ESTEEM

He who has to regularly escape

from his own reality,

needs to put more time and effort

into improving that reality.

If he is to ever escape from the

negative cycle of dysfunction

that he has now trapped himself in.

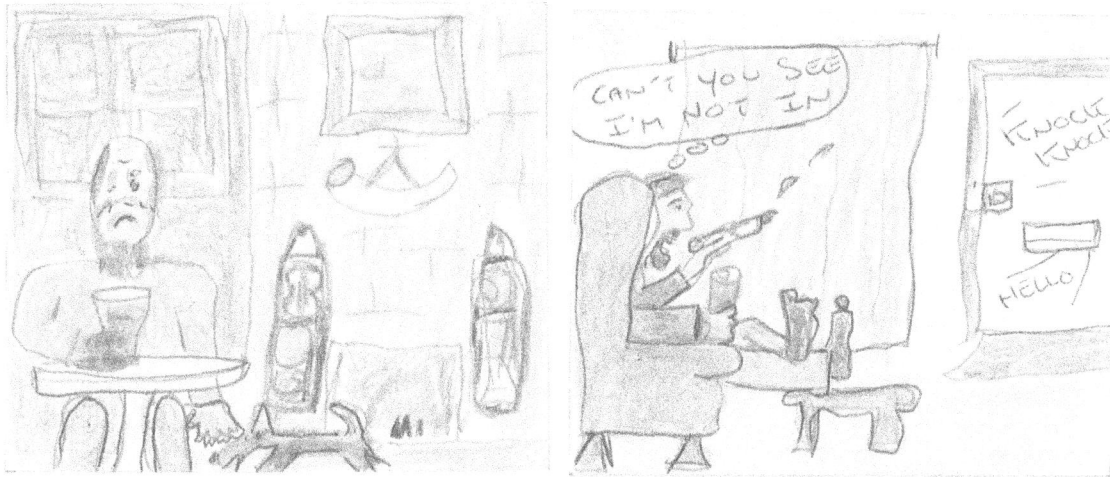

| Drugs and alcohol can often act as a depressant. | We can become withdrawn, anti-social and de-motivated. |

THE LINK BETWEEN DRUG AND ALCOHOL USE AND DEPRESSION.

There is a very strong link between drug and alcohol use and depression. We often feel that when we are low in mood we need some kind of stimulant to help us to forget our worries and to have a good time. Unfortunately most stimulants tend to actually exaggerate our problems and so when we are intoxicated or stoned, we are unable to tackle any problems in a rational manner. The situation becomes more and more hopeless and frustrating.

It has long been known that high alcohol intake can have a depressant after effect, but recent studies also suggest that most street drugs, if taken on a regular basis, can also have a long-term depressive effect. We can become withdrawn, anti-social and de-motivated. We can experience short-term memory difficulties, flashbacks and sever concentration problems. Physically we can experience increased aches and pains, hot sweats, shaking limbs, a lack of energy, poor diet and nutrition along with disturbed sleeping patterns. Socially we may become poor and isolated, often ending up living in conditions of severe depravation.

Now do Exercise 113.

165

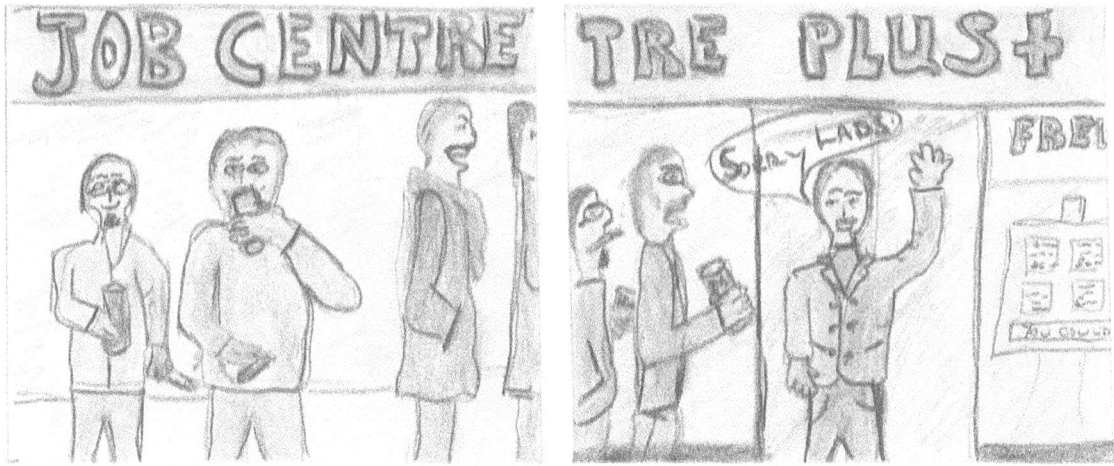

| Lots of people take drugs or alcohol to escape from reality. | Unfortunately this just makes reality far worse for them. |

WHY USE DRUGS AND ALCOHOL?

A lot of people try and use drugs or alcohol to escape from their problems because it can offer them a carefree role away from the stresses and strains of everyday life. Just how effective is it? The answer to that is, have you ever met anyone who has managed to get their life back on track by drinking too much or by taking drugs? Has anybody with a drugs or alcohol addiction ever struck you as somebody who has got his or her life totally sorted out? Do they ever strike you as people who know where they are going in life? It is not very likely that they do because the reality is that by trying to escape from your problems in this manner, you merely create far more problems that are often even more serious than the problems you started off with.

Never be fooled into thinking that getting drunk or stoned is the answer to all of your problems, it is not. It solves nothing and destroys everything. Going out for the odd drink with friends can often do us some good. Nobody is saying that you should not enjoy yourself. It is when it becomes the only way that you can enjoy yourself that you need to get things into perspective.

Now do Exercise 114.

166

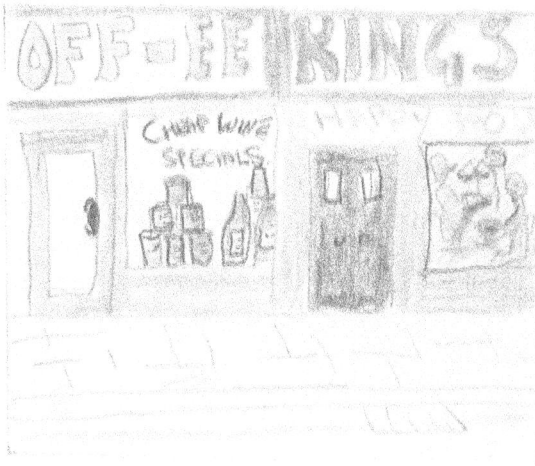

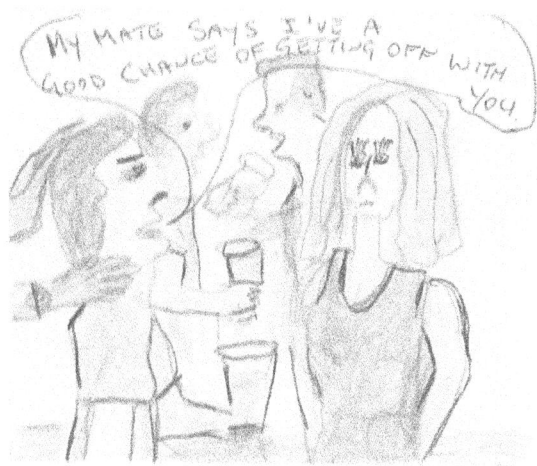

Is alcohol the legal drug of our time?	Young people use it to give themselves extra confidence.

THE SOCIAL EFFECTS OF ALCOHOL.

Alcohol is the accepted drug in our society. It is sold in every corner shop, public house and supermarket throughout the land. Glossy advertisements for it fill our magazines and television screens. The message that we get from society is that drinking is a good thing to do, but is it really any better than taking street drugs that are looked down upon by society? If you ask a drug and alcohol team worker, which is the greater problem, they will undoubtedly say that they receive many more referrals for alcohol-related problems than they do for drug-related problems. Alcohol dependency is as dangerous as any street drug dependency and is far more widespread.

Most people do drink alcohol and it is considered to be normal and socially acceptable. Young adults tend to go through a phase of drinking too much alcohol; this is because it breaks down any inhibitions and gives them a renewed sense of confidence and if they make a fool of themselves they can always blame it on the alcohol. Unfortunately some people have an addictive personality and so when they drink alcohol they can find it very difficult to stop.

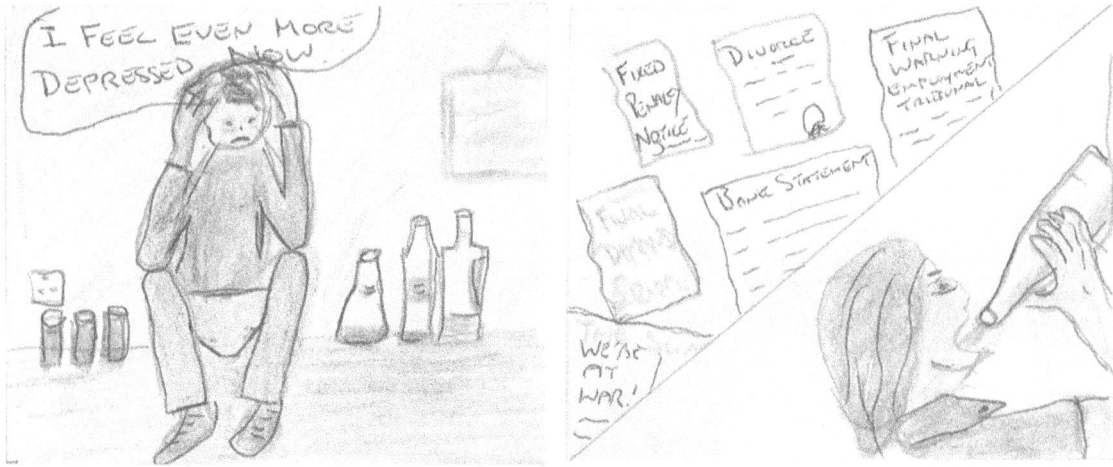

Alcohol enhances the feelings that we have already got.	Being drunk can feel safer than facing the true reality of your life.

WHAT DOES ALCOHOL DO TO US?

Alcohol can provide us with another role to escape into when our real world is becoming increasingly difficult to deal with. From our past experience getting drunk is usually associated with having a good time. In reality most of the times that we got drunk would have been happy occasions anyway, birthday, parties, etc. The alcohol only enhanced those happy feelings. Alcohol is however a depressant, so if we drink it because we are feeling sad or angry, it will only increase the intensity of these feelings. This is why you often see drunken people arguing or fighting; their inhibitions are decreased but their susceptibility to anger has increased, making them potentially very volatile.

Alcoholics are people who get stuck into this role of constantly being drunk. Like people stuck in the sick role, they tend to find it the safest place to be. As time goes by all of the other roles tend to have been badly affected and diminished by the alcoholic role, which will in turn make it feel even more desirable to stay in the alcoholic role. This is why alcoholics find it so difficult to break out of the drinking spiral. It will take a lot of effort to get all the other areas of their life back together again.

Now do Exercise 115.

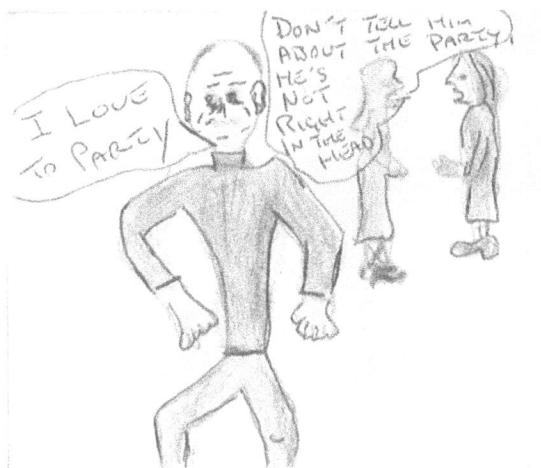

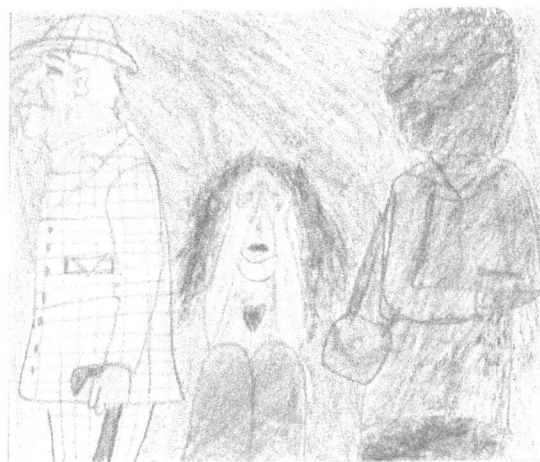

Alcoholics cause a lot of damage to themselves, both physically and mentally.	People will avoid you as your life starts to fall apart.

WHAT ARE THE DANGERS OF ALCOHOL ABUSE?

Alcohol can cause severe physical, social and mental damage. Physically it can damage your liver and stomach lining, decrease your eyesight, ruin your teeth, make you smell and it can be the underlying cause of numerous other physical conditions such as diabetes, impotency and obesity. Excessive drinking can also quite literally kill you!

Socially drinking can destroy all of your relationships; people will no longer trust you or believe in you, in fact they will probably do their best to avoid you. You will eventually become unemployable and a social outcast. Your appearance will start to deteriorate as you become more and more haggard looking and dejected. Mentally you run the risk of developing dementia or brain damage. You will become very repetitive, volatile and unpredictable. You may start to get visual or auditory hallucinations. You also run a high risk of becoming depressed as your life gradually starts to fall apart.

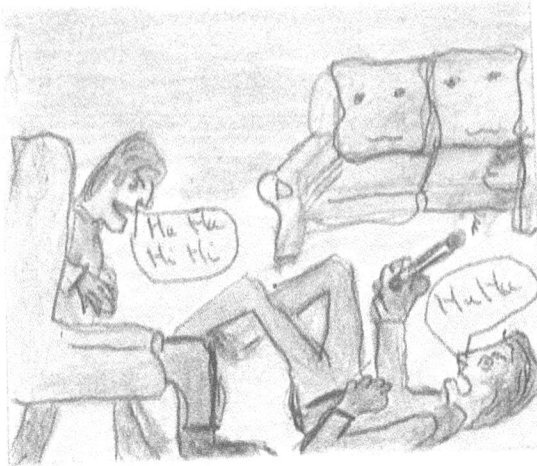

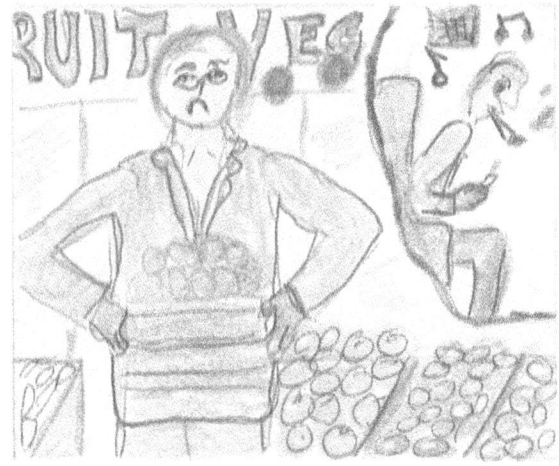

| Initial drug use can be enjoyable and good fun. | It can become a role that we use to hide in when reality becomes hard to cope with. |

WHY DO PEOPLE TAKE ILLEGAL DRUGS?

The main reason why people start to use street drugs is because they find the experience an enjoyable one. A number of factors may encourage somebody to start, including the availability, their own curiosity, the need to rebel, peer influence and peer pressure.

In the majority of cases drugs are offered to people by one of their close friends. This friend will have already enjoyed the experience and will be keen to share it. People continue to take drugs because they enjoy the effects that they have upon them. Being a drug user also offers the opportunity to develop a new role that can be fun and carefree, a role with no commitments or responsibility. This is very tempting to people who have problems that they would prefer to be able to forget. As reality becomes increasingly difficult for them to deal with, being in the drug user role appears to be a more attractive alternative. This is how drug dependency usually starts.

Now do Exercise 116.

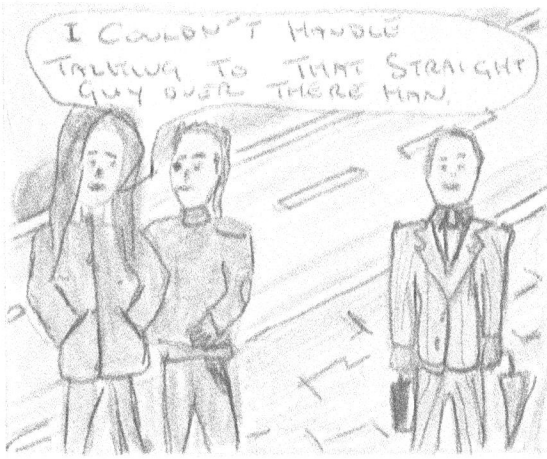

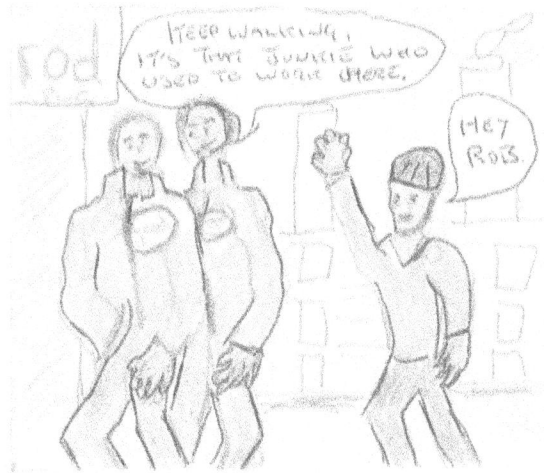

You start to only associate with other drug users.	You may lose your job and your real friends.

THE NEGATIVE SPIRAL OF DRUG USE.

As time goes on drug use increases because it seems to be the only way that you can have a good time. You start to only associate with other drug users because they are easier to relate to and other people don't understand you anyway. So all of your old friends gradually start to disappear. You start to become less motivated and so you give up past interests and hobbies in preference for more drug use. Money starts to become short as you miss days off work and have to fund your increasingly expensive habit. Crime can often become a very viable option. With a criminal record, no viable friends left that you can't trust and a poor work record, securing employment is going to be difficult. So now you have a lot more time on your hands, reality is miserable and depressing so you take more drugs to escape from it. This is a common picture for most dependent drug users. People don't have to remain stuck in this spiral, but unless they can manage to give up taking the drugs, it will be a very difficult pattern to break.

Now do Exercise 117.

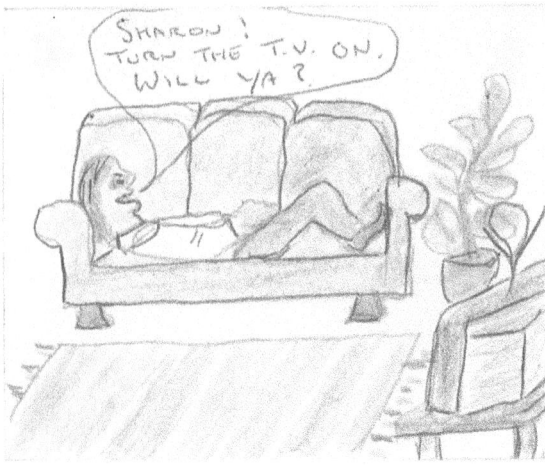

Cannabis users can suffer from a severe lack of energy.	They can become easily confused and anxious.

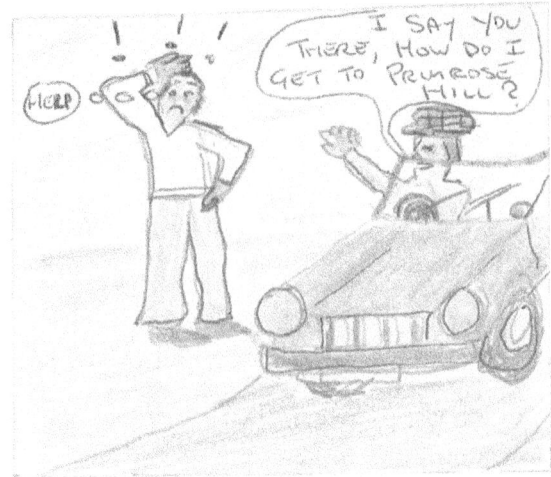

CANNABIS AND MENTAL HEALTH.

Cannabis is probably the most widely used street drug. Common effects include a pleasurable state of relaxation, talkativeness, bouts of hilarity, and increased sensory awareness. As with alcohol, the effects depend largely upon the users' expectations and their current state of mind. Cannabis is not addictive, although regular users may feel a psychological need for it.

The risks involved with cannabis use include: lack of energy, lethargy, forgetfulness, poor short-term memory, poor concentration, confused states, anxiety states, low self-esteem, lack of assertiveness and confidence, over-eating and increased susceptibility of psychotic episodes.

The effects of regular cannabis use can mimic the symptoms that we see in depression. Add this to the fact that regular cannabis users tend to cut themselves off from non-users and that they no longer have the energy and motivation to pursue any interests away from cannabis smoking and your start to realise how easy it is to become depressed when you regularly smoke cannabis.

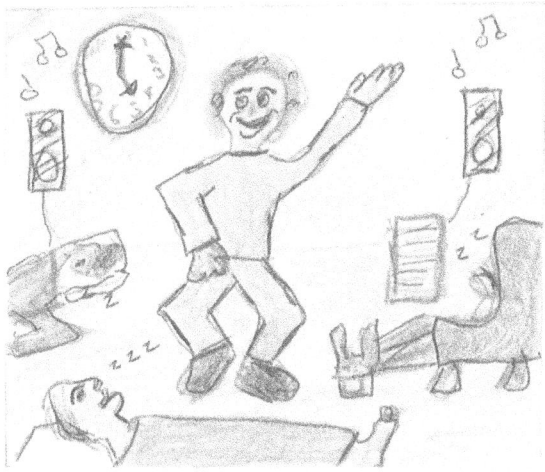

| Amphetamines make you feel very energetic and alert. | Prolonged use can cause physical and psychological damage. |

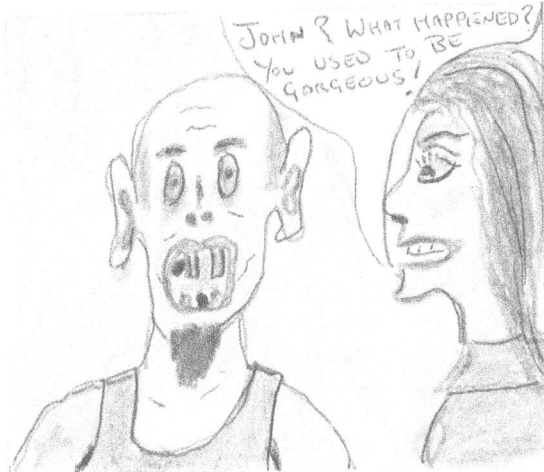

AMPHETAMINES AND MENTAL HEALTH.

Amphetamines, such as speed, have the effect of making the user feel more alert, energetic and confident as well as increasing levels of arousal. With high doses the user can experience feelings of intense exhilaration, a rapid flow of ideas, along with feelings of increased physical strength and greater mental capacity. These feelings can go on to produce feelings of panic, with hallucinations and paranoia, otherwise known as a drug-induced psychotic episode.

Long-term amphetamine use can also lead to severe weight loss, poor teeth, heart problems, sleep problems, social withdrawal, flashbacks and depression. There is also a risk that whoever you buy the amphetamine off will more than likely be unscrupulous and could start mixing the amphetamine with other substances in order to increase their profit. The user could then be at risk from consuming cut glass, soap powder or any number of dangerous compounds.

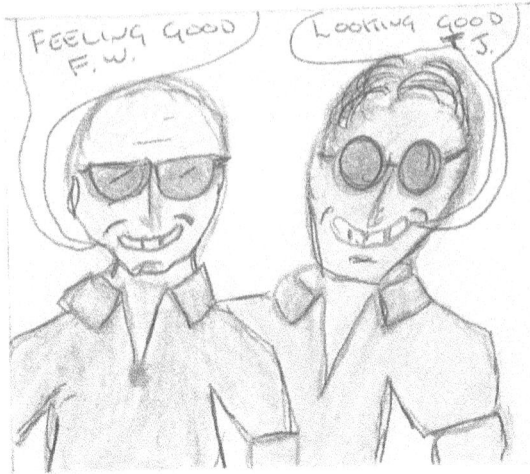

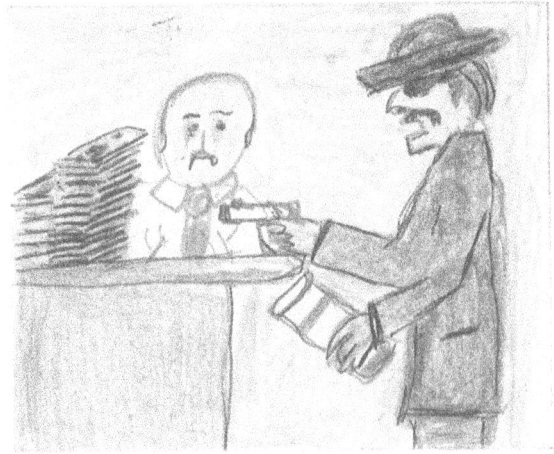

Cocaine is highly addictive due to its effect of euphoria.	Financing a cocaine habit could lead you into a life of crime.

COCAINE AND MENTAL HEALTH.

Cocaine tends to have a similar effect to amphetamines, but it is more extreme and short lived, hence the reason why it is so highly addictive. Its effects of contentment and euphoria are also very addictive as this is how most of us long to feel. Unfortunately there is a downside to cocaine use. It can make users feel chronically nervous, over-excitable and paranoid. Users can suffer sleep deprivation leading to feelings of confusion and restlessness, which in turn can lead to a state of paranoid psychosis. Physically users can suffer from weight loss, nausea and nasal damage. Cocaine is also a very expensive drug. Becoming addicted to it will need funding and this can lead to sever financial problems along with the temptation to get involved in criminal behaviour in order to finance your drug habit.

Cocaine use can clearly lead us down a very slippery slope that is more than likely going to result in us suffering from depression.

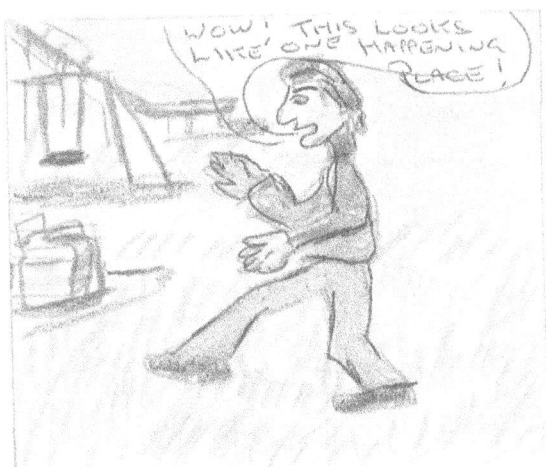

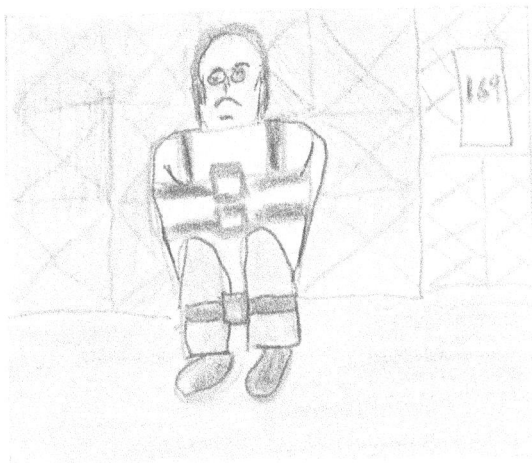

| Ecstasy heightens perception and produces a stimulating effect. | The psychological damage caused appears to be irreversible. |

ECSTASY AND MENTAL HEALTH.

Ecstasy is an amphetamine-based drug, which heightens perception and produces a stimulant effect. Prolonged use can cause anxiety, panic, confusion, insomnia and possibly psychosis.

The long-term effects of ecstasy use are still not yet fully known but there is a growing concern that the mental damage caused by the drug could well be permanent and irreversible. That means that a lot of today's ecstasy users will be tomorrow's long-term psychiatric patients!

Ecstasy can also bring up repressed feelings and emotions, which in turn can cause the user a lot of emotional turmoil and trauma. This can lead to either a psychotic breakdown or an episode of depression.

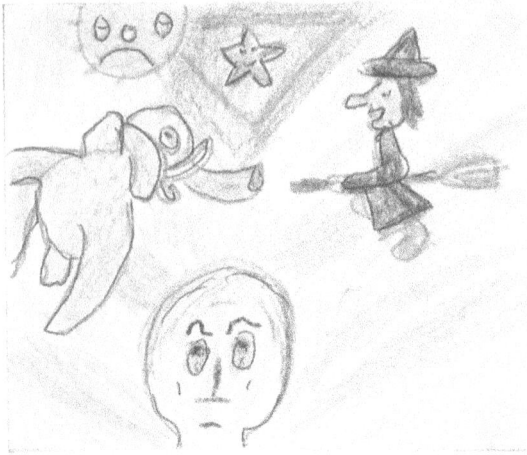

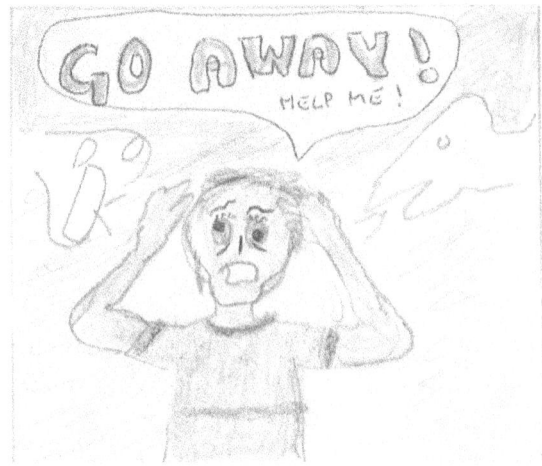

| LSD has a hallucinogenic effect. | It can easily push you into a psychotic episode. |

LSD (ACID) AND MENTAL HEALTH.

LSD is a hallucinogenic drug that can cause distortion to the users' perception of shapes and sizes, movement of objects, distortion of hearing and changes of time and place. Colours can appear more intense or psychedelic; experiences can seem mystical or distorted from reality. Some users feel dissociated from their own body. Unpleasant trips or experiences tend to happen more when the user is feeling anxious or depressed. Possible reactions include dizziness, depression, disorientation, short-lived psychotic episodes, hallucinations and paranoia.

Repeated use can produce prolonged serious psychological reactions. Some people suffer from flashbacks for many years after taking LSD. Flashbacks can be very distressing and may well lead to further psychiatric difficulties.

Now do Exercise 118.

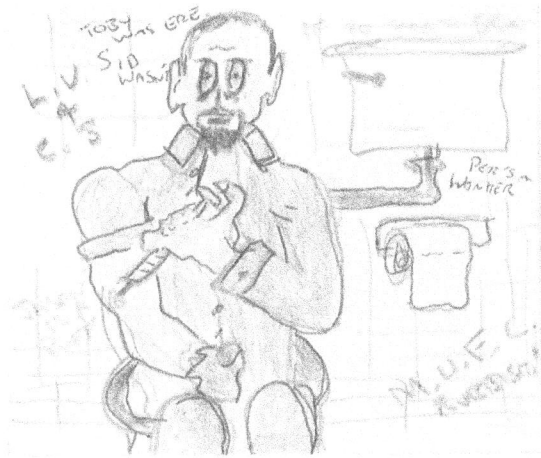

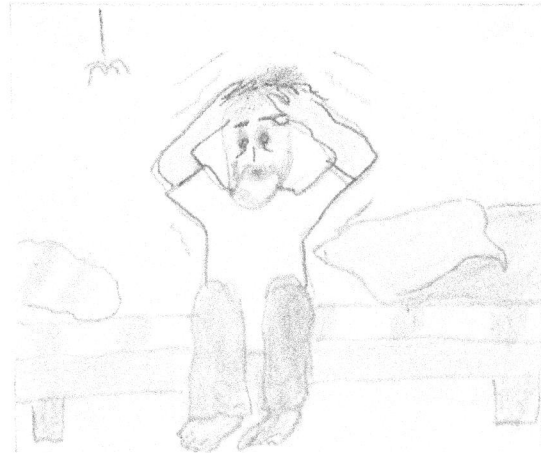

Heroin users soon develop tolerance, so they have to increase the amount that they take.	Withdrawal can be a very drawn out and painful process.

HEROIN AND MENTAL HEALTH.

Heroin can be sniffed smoked or injected. At lower levels it can produce a feeling of euphoria without affecting general functioning. At higher levels the user becomes drowsy and contented. Tolerance develops with regular use, so that to produce the same effect, higher doses and more immediate methods of administration must be used.

There does come a point when further increases only enable the user to feel normal, and stopping suddenly brings on withdrawal symptoms that are similar in effect to influenza and can last for several months. Long-term use of heroin can lead to decreased appetite, poor hygiene, apathy and consequent physical and mental health problems

Heroin also tends to destroy users' personalities; they can become very emotionless and almost shark-like in their lack of facial expressions. Another major problem for heroin users is funding their habit. Heroin can be very expensive and the people who sell it are generally not the sort of people that you want to owe money to! Heroin can therefore, also lead to a life of crime and depression.

Now do Exercise 119.

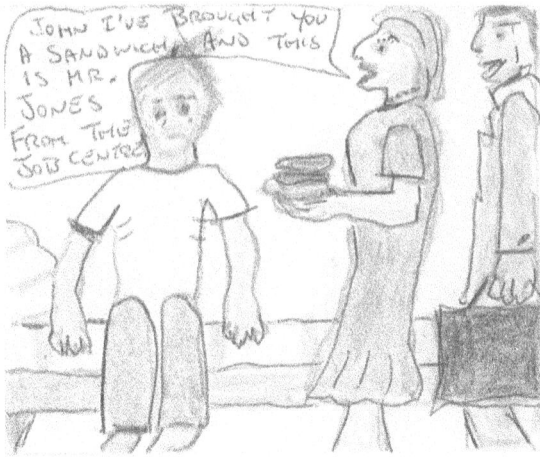

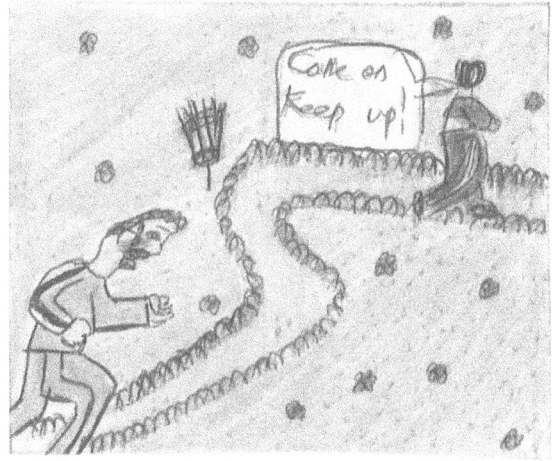

Let them know that you care about them and that you don't want to see them ruin their lives.	Encourage them to lead a healthy lifestyle.

WHAT CAN FAMILY AND FRIENDS DO TO HELP?

It is heartbreaking to see somebody that you know and love develop a drug addiction. So what is the best approach that you can adopt to help them? Firstly don't blame yourself, only the drug user can make the decision to quit, not you. Let them know that you love and care about them and that you find their drug habit very upsetting and destructive. Set clear limits to let them know that you are not prepared to permit drug taking to take place in your home. Encourage them to take part in some healthy activities and pursuits with you that are far removed from the world of drugs. Explain to them that other users are not their real friends and the only common bond that they have together is a shared drug habit. Encourage them to spend more time with real friends. Try and persuade them to stick to a healthy regular diet, along with a consistent routine.

Try to encourage them to talk about their problems rather than to cover them up with drugs. Above all be strong and try to remain optimistic that one day they will decide to quit.

SELF-HELP EXERCISES

CONQUERING DEPRESSION

EXERCISE 1.

Do you fit into any of the high-risk groups? If so how has it affected you?

Example: Being brought up in a poor family has made me feel unequal.

EXERCISE 2.

Have you started to neglect any tasks recently due top feelings of depression?

Example: I am not washing as regularly as I used to.

EXERCISE 3.

Write down a list of people who seem to be avoiding you, what happened the last time that you saw them?

Example: I didn't say a word to John the last time that he called around to see me.

EXERCISE 4.

Keep a record or how many hours sleep you are getting, is it increasing or decreasing?

Monday	Tuesday	Wednesday	Thursday	Friday	Saturday	Sunday
Hours	Hours	Hours	Hours	Hours	Hours	Hours

EXERCISE 5.

Keep a record of everything that you eat so that you can monitor your daily intake.

	Monday	Tuesday	Wednesday	Thursday	Friday	Saturday	Sunday
Breakfast							
Snacks between meals							
Lunch							
Snacks between meals							
Dinner							

EXERCISE 6.

How have your emotions recently changed?

Example: I cry a lot more than I used to.

EXERCISE 7.

How many hours a day are you sat just focusing on how depressed you have become?

Example: Monday sat in the chair for two hours in the morning, three hours in the afternoon.

Time	Monday	Tuesday	Wednesday	Thursday	Friday	Saturday	Sunday
9am							
10am							
11am							
12pm							
1pm							
2pm							
3pm							
4pm							
5pm							
6pm							
7pm							
8pm							
9pm							
10pm							
11pm							

EXERCISE 8.

Make a list of any new physical complaints that you have.

Example: Rash on my neck, painful knees.

EXERCISE 9.

Are you re-living past experiences over and over in your mind? Try viewing them from a fresh perspective.

Example: Those kids that picked on me at school had no idea what they were really doing they were only 10 years old at the time!

EXERCISE 11.

If you are experiencing visual or auditory hallucinations, try to describe them in as much detail as possible.

Example: A male voice inside my head keeps telling me to harm myself.

EXERCISE 12.

If you are experiencing suicidal thoughts make a list of help numbers that you can contact. Try to avoid being alone as much as possible. Write down exactly what you thoughts are so that you can challenge them.

Example: I feel worthless and unlovable.

Challenge: My friends like me and my mother always loved me, I can't be that bad.

EXERCISE 13.

Buy yourself a diary today!

EXERCISE 14.

Make an appointment with your GP to discuss the symptoms of your depression.

EXERCISE 15.

Construct a circle that shows how your symptoms all fuel each other.

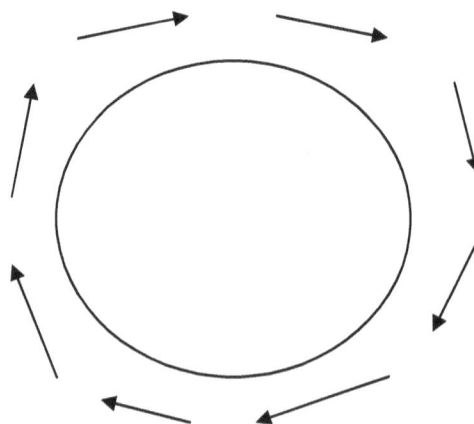

EXERCISE 16.

Do you really want to be depressed for the rest of your life?

Example: No

Do you want to lead a full and active life?

Example: Yes

Are you prepared to put in the effort required to get better?

Example: Yes.

EXERCISE 17.

List all of the changes that you would hope to see in yourself if you managed to conquer depression?

Example: More light hearted/easy going/relaxed/outgoing/assertive/confident.

EXERCISE 18.

Construct a list of your own personal beliefs.

Example: Equal rights/ animal rights, abortion laws/ religious views/ political opinions.

EXERCISE 19.

Now put these beliefs in order of importance to you.

1.

2.

3.

EXERCISE 20.

Write out a list of the things that you value.

Example: Time with my children/a good music system/ time to play golf.

EXERCISE 21.

List all of your interests then tick the ones that you are still actively involved with.

Example: Swimming/Tennis/Fishing+/Walking+/Painting/Kung fu/ Gliding.

EXERCISE 22.

Complete the following table on past, present and future interests. Tick the activities that you used to do in the past column, the activities you do now in the present column, and the activities that you hope to be doing in the future, in the future column.

Activity	Past	Present	Future
Artistic			
Sport/Health			
Club Member			
Sociable			
Educational			
Religious			
Helping others			
Travel			
Exhibitions			
Theatre			
Cinema			
Dance			
Gardening			
DIY			
Cooking			
Any other			

EXERCISE 23.

Write down a definite start date that you can realistically stick to.

DATE:

EXERCISE 24.

List the skills that you are currently struggling with:

Example: Hand eye co-ordination/memory/concentration

Now try to match these skills up to activities that use them:

Example: Pottery = hand eye co-ordination / concentration / planning / imagination /sequencing.

Cookery = Planning, time management / preparation / co-ordination / hand eye co-ordination / following instructions / sequencing.

EXERCISE 25.

Time	Monday	Tuesday	Wednesday	Thursday	Friday	Saturday	Sunday
7am							
8am							
9am							
10am							
11am							
12pm							
1pm							
2pm							
3pm							
4pm							
5pm							
6pm							
7pm							
8pm							
9pm							
10pm							
11pm							

Construct a simple timetable.

EXERCISE 26.

Set yourself a start date from when you intend to use your timetable.

DATE:

EXERCISE 27.

List some of the roles you currently take on.

Example: I am assertive as a parent but not as a customer.

EXERCISE 28.

Complete the following roles table.

Roles	Past	Present	Future
Student			
Volunteer			
Caregiver			
Home Maintainer			
Friend			
Parent			
Son/Daughter			
Brother/Sister			
Husband/Wife			
Religious Participant			
Sporting participant			
Sporting Spectator			
Teacher of skills			
Learner of skills			
Hobbyist			
Participant in an organisation			
Any others			

EXERCISE 29.

Identify which roles you function the best in and make plans to increase the amount of time that you spend in those roles.

Example: I am confident, relaxed and happy at the golf club, I need to increase the amount of time that I spend there.

EXERCISE 30.

Write down as many ideas as you can for possible long-term goals.

Example: Walk the Andes / Learn to drive/ build a matchstick model of the Eiffel tower.

EXERCISE 31.

Once you have decided upon your long-term goal, work out some short-term goals to help you get there.

Example: Long-term goal = Walk the Andes.

Short term   Goal (1) = Start walking every weekend.

Goal (2) = walk 3 times a week.

Goal (3) = Walk 12 miles every other day. Etc.

EXERCISE 32.

Return to exercise 5. How could you improve your diet?

Example: cut down on crisps and chocolate and eat fruit between meals instead.

EXERCISE 33.

Spend some time recording your favourite feel good pieces of music.

EXERCISE 34.

Go to your local library and arrange to hire out a funny film.

EXERCISE 35.

Make some positive plans to do more exercise.

Example: I am going to start swimming on Mondays and Thursday.

EXERCISE 36.

My treatment plan for conquering depression.

Using all of the information from the past 35 exercises answer as many of the following questions as you can.

1) My depression seems to be caused by

   ………………………………………………………………………

2) Things that are likely to make my depression worse

   ………………………………………………………………………

3) I can make my life better by

   ………………………………………………………………………

4) I intend to start doing things that I want to do like

   ………………………………………………………………………

5) I intend to improve my physical fitness by

   ………………………………………………………………………

6) I intend to improve my mental fitness by

   ………………………………………………………………………

7) I shall improve my inner harmony by using my values and beliefs to guide my actions by ……………………………………………………………………

8) My long-term goal is

   ………………………………………………………………………

9) I shall improve my social life by

   ………………………………………………………………………

10) I promise myself that I shall do everything possible to combat depression……………………………………………………………………

    ………………………………………………………………

CONQUERING ANXIETY

EXERCISE 37.

Write down any symptoms that might be acting as a bridge between anxiety and depression.

Example: I feel anxious because I always expect that something bad is about to happen to me.

EXERCISE 38.

List all of the physical symptoms that you experience when you feel anxious

Example: Hear racing/short breaths/stomach pains etc.

EXERCISE 39.

List all of the places and people that you have recently been avoiding due to your anxious feelings.

Example: The post office / the supermarket /the next door neighbour, etc.

EXERCISE 40.

Recall some previous anxiety attacks, did you make them worse by thinking negatively? Are you creating your own anxiety spiral?

EXERCISE 41.

Have you developed any new habits or rituals in order to avoid getting anxious? What are they?

Example: I check the car door 10 times.

EXERCISE 42.

Identify what you really fear might happen to you.

Example: I might be humiliated / people might laugh at me.

EXERCISE 42.

List the things that you are now going to do to help you relax.

Example: Listen to relaxing music daily / have a country walk twice a week, etc.

EXERCISE 44.

Choose two situations from exercise 39 that you would really like to change. Now put together some short-term goals to help you to achieve them.

1.

2.

EXERCISE 45.

Set a start date for beginning exercise 44.

EXERCISE 46.

List as many of your regular negative thoughts as possible.

Example: Everybody stares at me / I always say something foolish.

EXERCISE 47.

Counteract the negative thoughts with positive ones.

Example:

Negative thought – this is an awful run down looking town.

Positive thought - It does have very good facilities like a large library and swimming pool.

CONQUERING STRESS.

EXERCISE 48.

Write down the times in the day that seem to increase your stress levels. Why do you think this is?

Example: Driving to work always upsets me.

EXERCISE 49.

Write down three lists in order to understand your stress levels better.

List 1:Tasks that I find boring

List 2:Tasks that I find stressful.

List 3:Tasks that I find interesting and rewarding.

EXERCISE 50.

List some situations when you became over stressed. Do you think that you would have achieved a better outcome by remaining calm?

Example: I shouted at the next-door neighbour for playing his music too loud.

Result: We are no longer on speaking terms.

EXERCISE 51.

Write down the symptoms that have affected you through being stressed.

Example: Increased chest pains / poor sleep.

EXERCISE 52.

List some of the things that are currently causing you to feel stressed.

Example Too many changes at work / lack of finance.

EXERCISE 53.

List some of the tasks that you have had to learn in the past in order to adapt.

Example I had to learn how to keep records on a computer at work.

EXERCISE 54.

Have you ever had to perform a task without adequate time to prepare for it? How did it make you feel?

EXERCISE 55.

Look at exercise 52 again and try using the brainstorming technique in order to look at possible alternative approaches.

EXERCISE 56.

Construct a weekly timetable that allows for a balanced lifestyle.

Time	Monday	Tuesday	Wednesday	Thursday	Friday	Saturday	Sunday
8am	Breakfast						
9am	Work						
10am	Coffee						
11am	Work						
12pm	Work						
1pm	Swimming						
2pm	Lunch						
3pm	Work						
4pm	Work						
5pm	Work						
6pm	Dinner						
7pm	Badminton						
8pm	Think						
9pm	TV						
10pm							

EXERCISE 57.

Now add an hour slot for thinking each day, make sure that it fits in well with the rest of your day and that you will not be interrupted.

EXERCISE 58.

Make some definite plans to start a new sport on a regular basis. Add it to your timetable.

EXERCISE 59.

Hire out a funny film or book. Make time for enjoyment and laughter in your life.

EXERCISE 60.

Has anything changed about your bedtime routine? What did you used to do? Try sticking to a healthy regular nighttime routine.

Example: Hot chocolate at 10pm. Read in bed for one hour, then turn the light out.

EXERCISE 61.

Write down the changes that you need to make to your diet and your overall eating habits.

Example: I am going to eat my lunch away from the office everyday. I am going to stick to fruit between meals.

CONQUERING LOW SELF-ESTEEM.

EXERCISE 62.

Try and list five positive qualities about yourself.

Example: I am a good listener.

1.

2.

3.

4.

5.

EXERCISE 63.

If you managed to feel good about yourself what treat would you reward yourself with?

Example: A new suit / A new haircut / A massage.

EXERCISE 64.

Complete as many of the following statements as possible.

The think I like most about my appearance is my ....

My greatest skills are ....

I reckon that I am pretty good at ....

The hardest thing that I have ever accomplished is ....

The thing that I am most proud of in my life is ....

EXERCISE 65.

List five things that always make you feel better about yourself.

Example: A bubble bath / a long walk.

1.

2.

3.

4.

5.

EXERCISE 66.

Practice listening to your inner intuition, write down what it is saying to you.

Example: I should be doing a more rewarding job.

EXERCISE 67.

Write down a list of your strongly held beliefs, underline the ones that seem to be causing you some problems. Are those beliefs really worth holding onto?

EXERCISE 68.

List all of the negative messages that you are constantly giving yourself, and then challenge them with truthful positive statements.

I am always late.	I am occasionally late for work, but I am usually on time.

CONQUERING POOR ASSERTIVENESS.

EXERCISE 69.

List the difficulties that you currently have when it comes to behaving assertively.

Example: I am afraid of upsetting other people.

EXERCISE 70.

List any advantages that you can see in behaving passively.

EXERCISE 71.

Why do you think that some people end up choosing to behave passively?

EXERCISE 72.

List as many disadvantages as you can think of for behaving aggressively.

EXERCISE 73.

What effect do aggressive people tend to have upon you? Write down how they make you feel about yourself.

EXERCISE 74.

What do you think the disadvantages of behaving in an indirectly aggressive manner might be?

EXERCISE 75.

If you know anybody who is indirectly aggressive write down how you feel about his or her behaviour.

EXERCISE 76.

Try to list some situations when you think that being assertive might not be the best way to behave.

EXERCISE 77.

Write down some situations where you feel that it would be appropriate to invade somebody else's body space.

EXERCISE 78.

Write down the effect that different body gestures have upon you.

EXERCISE 79.

How do you feel about expressing your true feelings? Practice disclosing your true feelings with somebody that you trust and write down how it makes you feel.

EXERCISE 80.

Do you give out clear precise messages? Do you think that there is any room for improvement?

EXERCISE 81.

Are you able to express empathy towards other people? Practice empathising on a regular basis and write down how it changes situations for you.

EXERCISE 82.

How good are you at choosing the right moment to ask for what you want?
Practice asking people for things at various times in the day to see how the
response varies.

EXERCISE 83.

Are you prepared to compromise? Or do you try to win every situation?
Practice working towards a compromise with various different people and then
record how it makes you feel.

EXERCISE 84.

Construct a list of equal rights that you feel everyone should be entitled to
have.

Example: Freedom of speech / The right to make mistakes.

EXERCISE 85.

Do you ask yourself how you are feeling on a regular basis? Learn to
acknowledge, accept and if necessary express your true feelings. Then record
how you feel about doing it.

EXERCISE 86.

What do you find so difficult about saying no? Write down your fears and concerns.

EXERCISE 87.

Are you good at hiding your true feelings or does your body language tend to give a lot more away about you than you think?

EXERCISE 88.

Do you make direct requests or are you guilty of trying to get what you want by dropping hints? Practice making direct requests accepting the fact that others have the right to reject your request if they want to.

EXERCISE 89.

Does criticism tend to make you crumple? Get to know your own crumple buttons and learn to understand how and why they hurt so much.

EXERCISE 90.

How do you tend to deal with criticism? Which behaviour type do you become? Practice dealing with criticisms assertively and record how it makes you feel.

EXERCISE 91.

Do your arguments ever involve digging up old resentments? Regularly practice trying to get to the root cause of the disagreement and then working towards a resolution or a compromise. Always avoid becoming side tracked.

EXERCISE 92.

Practice criticising other people in an assertive manner and record how much better it feels compared to your old method.

EXERCISE 93.

How have society/s messages about our sexuality impacted upon your life?

Example: I could not pursue a career as a ballet dancer because it wasn't a masculine profession.

EXERCISE 94.

What changes do you now have to make in order to feel assertive?

CONQUERING ANGER.

EXERCISE 95.

How do you currently deal with your feelings of anger?

Mentally:

Physically:

Behaviourally:

EXERCISE 96.

Write down exactly why you think that you feel angry so often.

EXERCISE 97.

Could anything be done now to change that situation? Can you change the way that you view the situation so that it no longer possess the power to make you angry?

EXERCISE 98.

List all of the problems that your anger has caused you to date.

EXERCISE 99.

Do you ever go into rage behaviour? How does that make you feel about yourself? What problems does it cause?

EXERCISE 100.

Do you fear your own temper? What do you fear might happen?

EXERCISE 101.

Write down the situations that are most likely to produce an angry response in you. What is the first sensation that you experience?

EXERCISE 102.

Learn to recognise the physical sensations that you start to feel when you begin to get angry. Make a list of them.

EXERCISE 103.

Practice the quick relaxation technique on a regular basis, at least twice a day.

EXERCISE 104.

Does getting angry help you to reach the outcome that you want to achieve?

EXERCISE 105.

Are you regularly making the same thinking errors? List the errors that you often make.

Example: I am always expecting others to criticise me.

EXERCISE 106.

What things have the power to put you in a bad mood?

EXERCISE 107.

Do you think that the things that you have just listed in exercise 106 should be able to wield so much power over you or should you be able to override them?

EXERCISE 108.

Practice writing down your angry feelings in a way that helps you to understand them in more details.

1. Who am I angry with?

2. How angry do I feel?

3. Why has this made me angry?

EXERCISE 109.

Try to recall which roles you were in the last three times that you became angry. Are you prone to becoming angry in some roles more than others? Write down which roles you are most likely to become angry in.

EXERCISE 110.

What do you gain from losing your temper? Are you benefiting in any way from it?

Example: It makes people afraid of me so I don't get hassled.

EXERCISE 111.

Are you angry about the past? List some of the things that still play on your mind and make you feel angry. Then decide how else you might be able to remember those events. Can you lower their impact upon you? If you can't, would you be prepared to seek out counselling?

EXERCISE 112.

Do you become easily frustrated with yourself? If so, why? How could you change your approach to these things?

CONQUERING ALCOLHOL ADDICTION.

EXERCISE 113.

Do you share a lot of the symptoms of depression? List the symptoms that you tend to suffer from.

EXERCISE 114.

Keep a weekly diary of how much alcohol you consume so that you can see how much it is increasing or decreasing by. You can also use it to highlight how much you are spending on alcohol each week.

Day	Monday	Tuesday	Wednesday	Thursday	Friday	Saturday	Sunday
Amount	6 x pints of lager 3 x large gin and tonics. Total cost =£15						

EXERCISE 115.

Why do you think that you drink so much? Is it to escape from other problems or does it give you the confidence that you want? Make a list of your reasons for drinking/

CONQUERING DRUG ADDICTION.

EXERCISE 116.

Do you remember what tempted you to try drugs in the first place?

EXERCISE 117.

Have you become trapped into a negative cycle of drug taking in order to avoid the problems of reality?

EXERCISE 118.

Which drugs do you regularly take?

EXERCISE 119.

Are you experiencing any detrimental effects to?

   a) Your thinking?

   b) Your physical well being?

   c) Your behaviour?

   d) Your mood?

   e) Your mental health?

   f) Your personality?

   g) Your morality?

GETTING TO KNOW YOURSELF.

The following exercises are designed to help you to get to know yourself better.

EXERCISE 1.

List your 10 favourite films.

1

2

3

4

5

6

7

8

9

10

EXERCISE 2.

List your 10 favourite songs of all time.

1

2

3

4

5

6

7

8

9

10

EXERCISE 3.

List your 10 favourite meals of all time.

1

2

3

4

5

6

7

8

9

10

EXERCISE 4.

List your top 10 holiday destinations.

1

2

3

4

5

6

7

8

9

10

EXERCISE 5.

List 5 activities that you would really like to try at some point in your life.

1

2

3

4

5

Now use this information to successfully guide yourself into leading the sort of life that you will feel content with.

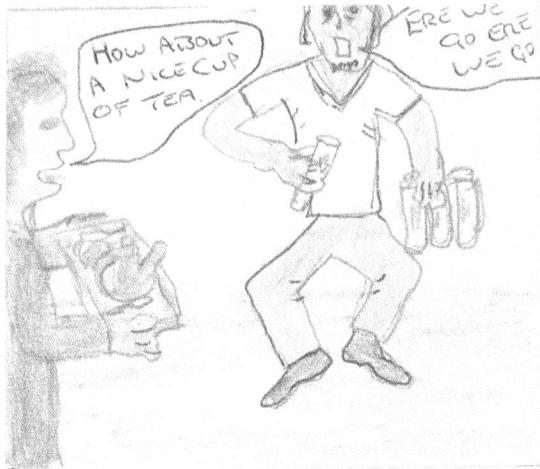

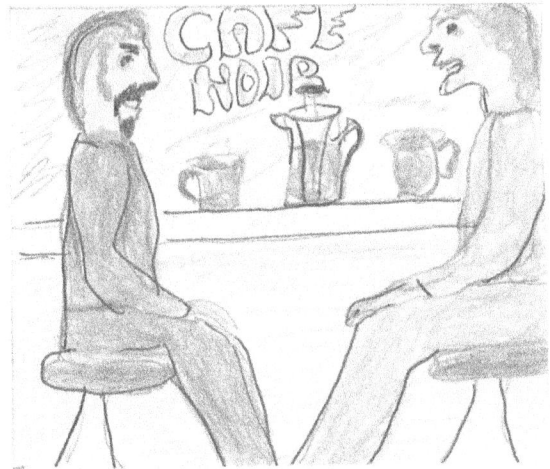

Do not allow their destructive behaviour to depress you.		Encourage them to discuss their difficulties with you.

WHAT CAN FAMILY AND FRIENDS DO TO HELP?

It is not easy to live with somebody who appears to be on a vary self-destructive course, if you are not careful it can start to bring you down as well, so it is always important to protect yourself from his or her destructive nature. Set clear boundaries, let them clearly know that you are not prepared to accept certain behaviours from them and spell out exactly what the consequences will be for them if they break any of these boundaries. What the boundaries are and what the consequences will be for breaking them can only ultimately be your decision. The only clear recommendation I can make is that you stick to your decision and carry out the threat that you have stated; otherwise they are soon going to learn that they can easily get around you.

Let them know that you love them and care about them, express how saddened you feel by their destructive behaviour, try to assist them in making other roles in their lives more valuable to them than the alcoholic role. Encourage them to engage in other more meaningful activities, allow them the opportunity to discuss their difficulties with you when they are sober and rational.

www.ingramcontent.com/pod-product-compliance
Lightning Source LLC
Chambersburg PA
CBHW080852300326
41935CB00041B/1549